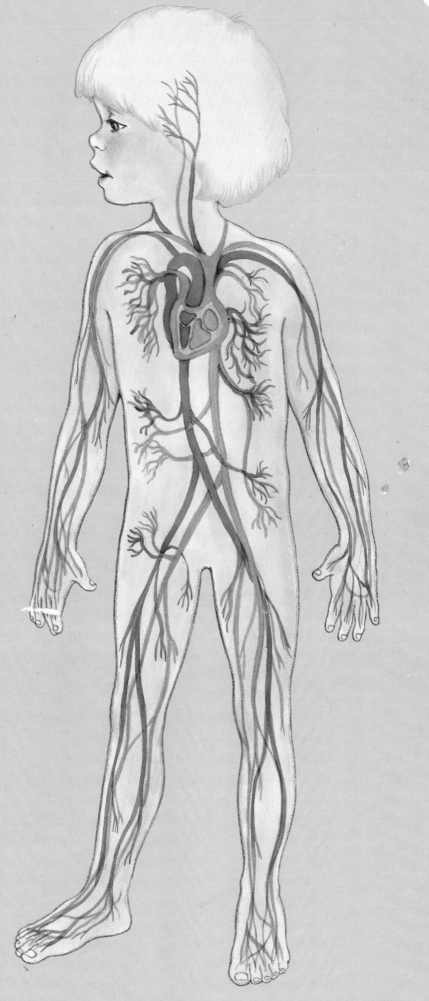

FROM HEAD TO TOES

How Your Body Works

by MARY PACKARD • Illustrated by DORA LEDER

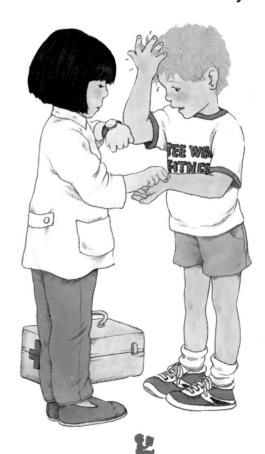

Little Simon
Published by Simon & Schuster, Inc., New York

A special thanks to Dr. Clifford M. Weingarten
for his careful review of my manuscript.

Library of Congress Cataloging in Publication Data

Packard, Mary.
    From Head to Toes. How Your Body Works

    Summary: Describes different parts of the body,
including the circulatory, digestive, nervous, and
reproductive systems, and explains how they work.
    1. Anatomy, Human—Juvenile literature.
2. Body, Human—Juvenile literature. [1. Anatomy,
Human. 2. Body, Human] I. Leder, Dora, ill. II. Title.
QM27.P25 1985   611   84-20163
ISBN 0-671-49772-3
       0-671-55750-5 (lib. bdg.)

Design by Antler & Baldwin Design Group

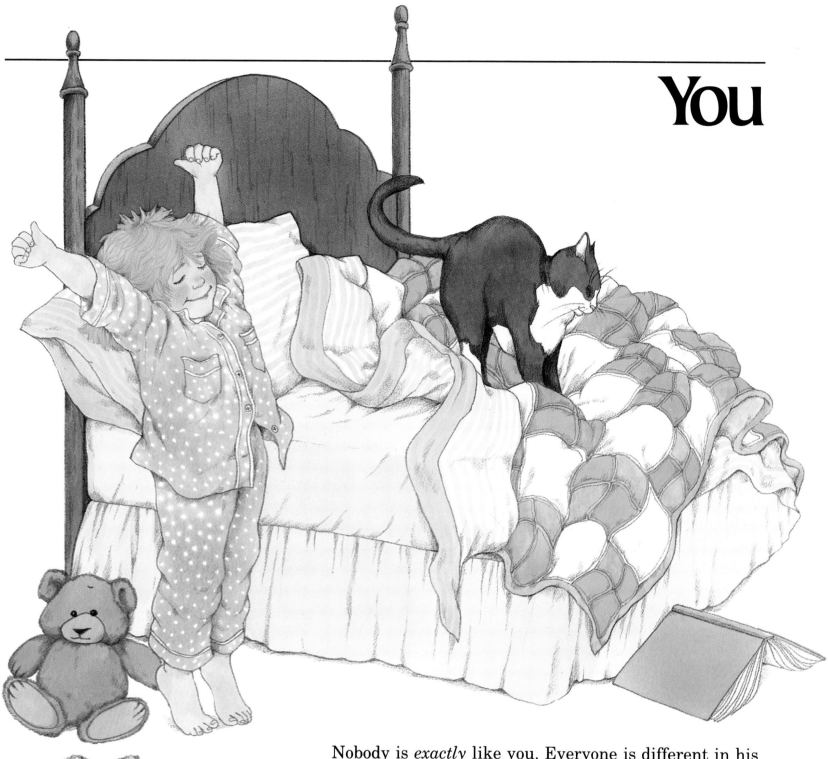

Stretching in the morning helps get your body ready for work again.

Nobody is *exactly* like you. Everyone is different in his or her own way. The way you smile, the twinkle in your eye, whatever makes you giggle—these are just some of the things that make you special.

The way the inside of your body works is very special, too. You can't see what's happening, but lots of interesting things are going on in there all the time. Let's look at some of the things that you might do during the day and find out how your body helps you do them.

Most of us start our mornings with a great big stretch. After we've been sleeping for a long time, stretching helps our muscles get ready for hard work again. But some of the muscles in our bodies never sleep. The heart is one of these muscles. Your heart is the strongest muscle in your body.

Heart, Blood, and Circulation

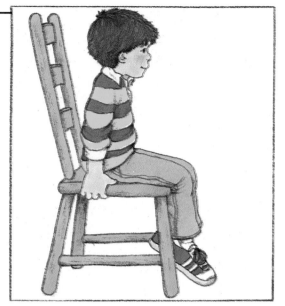

Your heart is the most frequently used muscle in your body. It is about the same size as your hand when you make a fist. Now open and close your fist. What you are doing is like the work your heart does every minute of the day and night. Squeeze, rest, squeeze, rest, thump, thump, thump. Sometimes your heart beats faster than it does other times. When you rest, your heart beats more slowly. After you've had a fast run, you can feel your heart pounding faster than usual in your chest.

Why does your heart have to work all of the time? Because it is your heart's job to push your blood all around the inside of your body. Every little part of you has its own job to do. And every little part needs the food and oxygen that are in your blood to keep on working. The muscles in your face need food and oxygen so you can smile. The muscles in your feet need food and oxygen in case you feel like wiggling your toes. Your eyes and ears need food and oxygen, too, so you can see and hear.

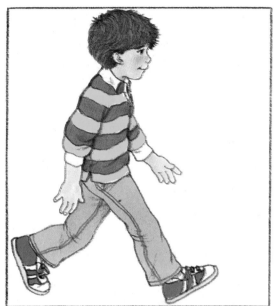

That incredible living pump called your heart pumps blood in a continuous cycle throughout your body. Your heart is divided into four parts or *chambers*. These chambers keep the blood without oxygen from getting mixed up with the blood that has oxygen. Each chamber has a little passageway, or *valve*, that shuts with a thump after blood enters. This keeps your blood from flowing back the other way. It is the closing of these valves that creates the thumping of your heart.

The two chambers of the right side of the heart are called the *right atrium* and the *right ventricle*. They take in used blood and send it to the lungs for more oxygen. The two chambers on the left are called the *left atrium* and *left ventricle*. They receive the fresh blood with oxygen from the lungs.

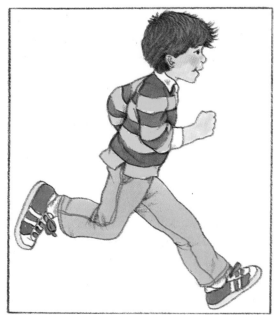

The more active you are, the faster your heart beats.

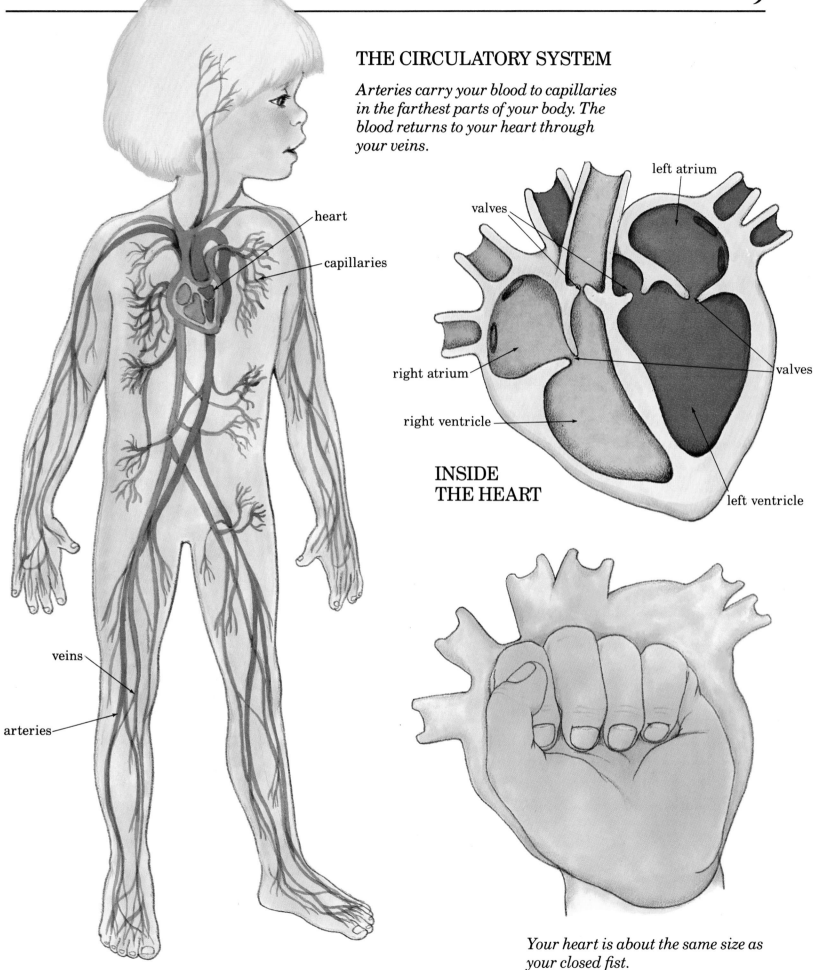

THE CIRCULATORY SYSTEM

Arteries carry your blood to capillaries in the farthest parts of your body. The blood returns to your heart through your veins.

heart

capillaries

left atrium

valves

right atrium

valves

right ventricle

left ventricle

INSIDE THE HEART

veins

arteries

Your heart is about the same size as your closed fist.

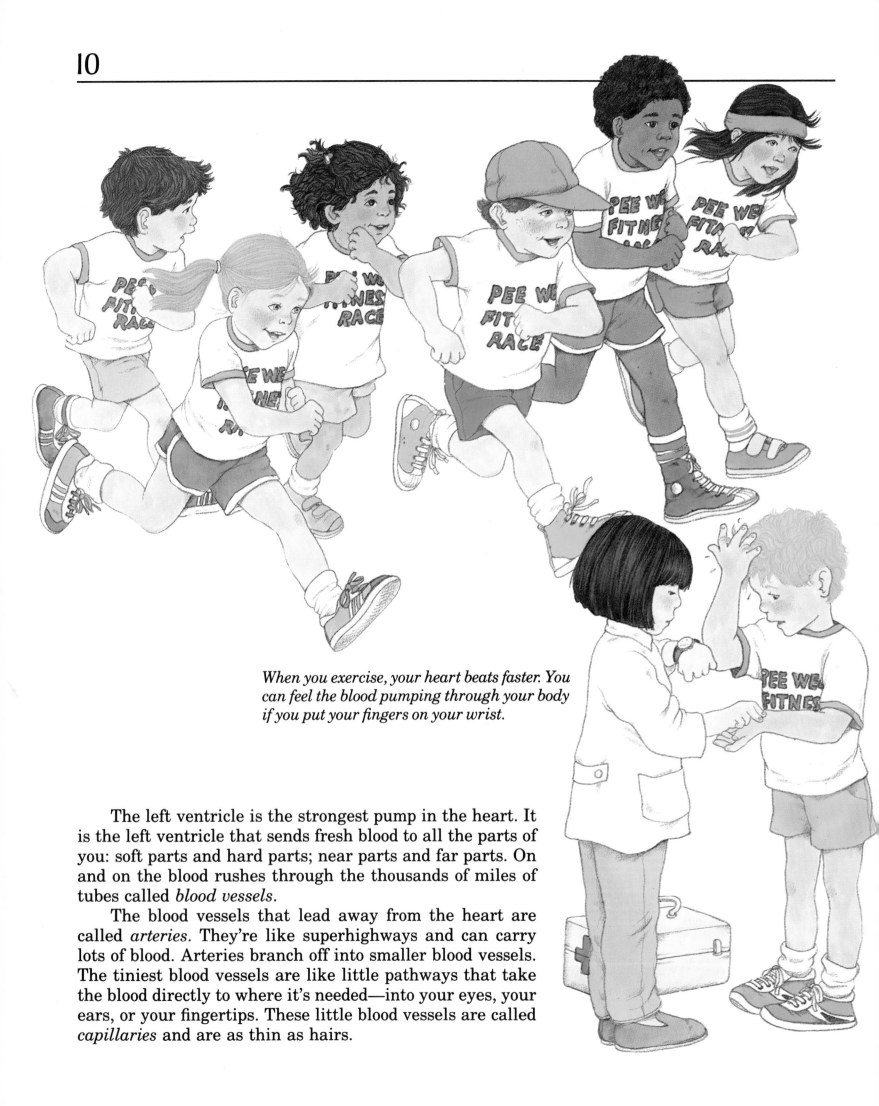

When you exercise, your heart beats faster. You can feel the blood pumping through your body if you put your fingers on your wrist.

The left ventricle is the strongest pump in the heart. It is the left ventricle that sends fresh blood to all the parts of you: soft parts and hard parts; near parts and far parts. On and on the blood rushes through the thousands of miles of tubes called *blood vessels*.

The blood vessels that lead away from the heart are called *arteries*. They're like superhighways and can carry lots of blood. Arteries branch off into smaller blood vessels. The tiniest blood vessels are like little pathways that take the blood directly to where it's needed—into your eyes, your ears, or your fingertips. These little blood vessels are called *capillaries* and are as thin as hairs.

HOW THE HEART PUMPS BLOOD

Your heart is a muscle that beats by contracting, just as if you were squeezing your fist. When the heart muscle relaxes, a valve in each atrium opens and blood floods into the ventricles. When the heart muscle contracts, new valves open and blood is pumped to your lungs through the pulmonary artery, and to the rest of your body through the aorta.

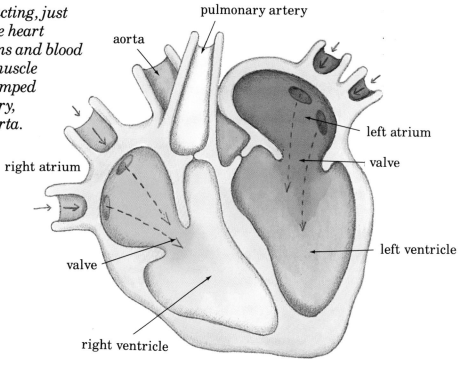

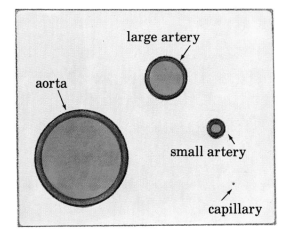

The closer the blood vessels are to your heart, the larger they are.

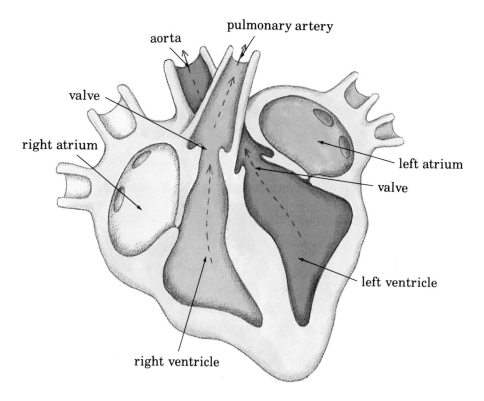

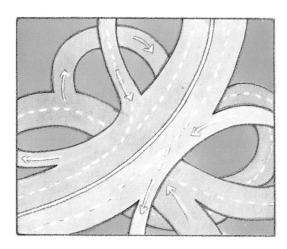

Arteries carrying blood from your heart to all parts of your body, and veins returning it to your heart, are like highways stretching through your body.

As the blood goes back to the heart, it empties from capillaries into larger and larger blood vessels called *veins*. The heart keeps your blood moving all of the time—and at a pretty fast pace, too. It only takes about one minute for a drop of blood to leave the heart, go down to your toe, and come all the way back again!

CROSS SECTION OF A BLOOD VESSEL

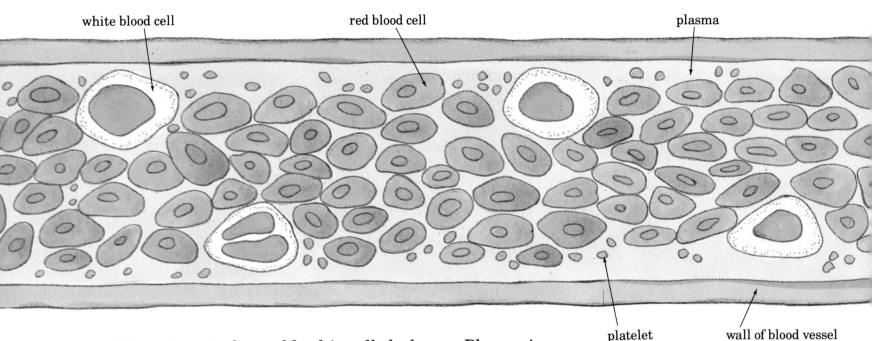

white blood cell   red blood cell   plasma

platelet   wall of blood vessel

The wet part of your blood is called *plasma*. Plasma is a yellowish liquid that is mostly water. Floating in the plasma are the other parts of your blood: little bits of digested food, *red blood cells, white blood cells,* and *platelets.* (Cells are very small, basic units of living matter. All living things are made of cells. Your body is made of many different types of cells.)

The red blood cells carry oxygen, which is the special life-giving part of air. Red blood cells are what give blood its red color.

White blood cells are another very important part of your blood. These special "germ eaters" kill harmful germs that may have found their way inside your body through your nose, your mouth, or through a cut. White blood cells rush to the spot where germs have landed and kill by swallowing them up.

Platelets help to heal your wounds. You may have noticed that when you get a cut, the blood doesn't keep on trickling out. It flows for a little while to wash away any dirt or germs. Then it slowly stops. That's because of special "blood savers" in the plasma called *fibrin* and *platelets.* Pieces of fibrin are like little threads that stick together and cover your cut like a spider's web. Platelets are tiny pieces broken from the red blood cells. They fill in the holes of the "spider's web" so that no more blood can leak out. Before long, the fibrin and platelets harden into a *scab.* The scab protects your cut so that no new germs can get into it. After your cut has mended, your scab falls off and your skin is as good as new again.

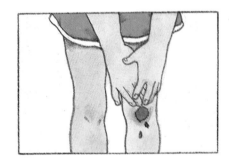

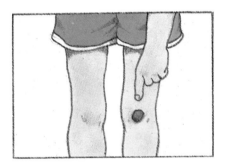

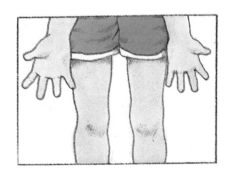

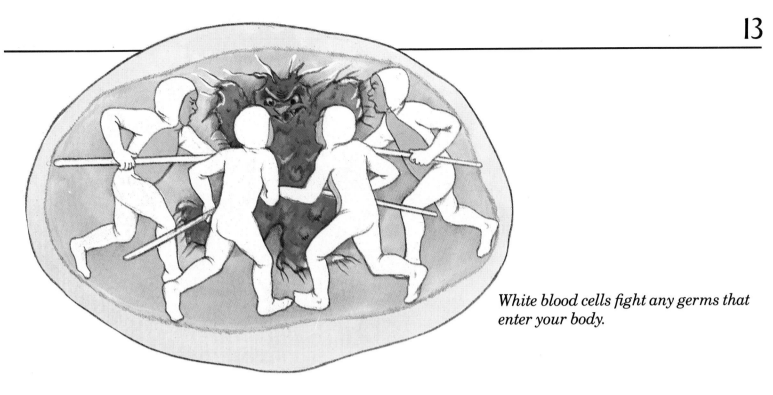

White blood cells fight any germs that enter your body.

If you scrape your knee, platelets form a scab that protects the cut from germs. The scab falls off when the cut is healed.

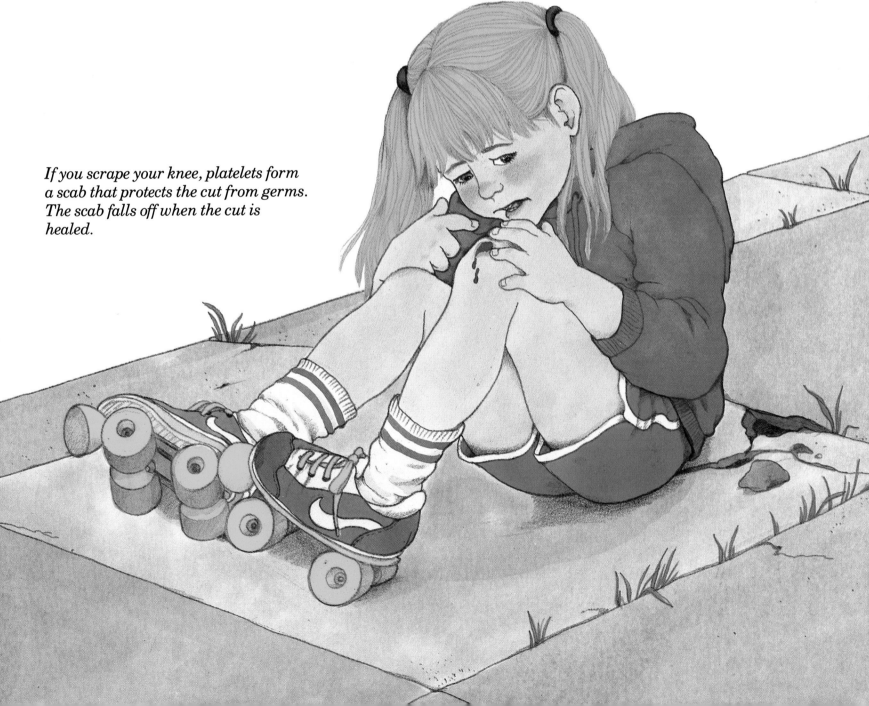

Skin

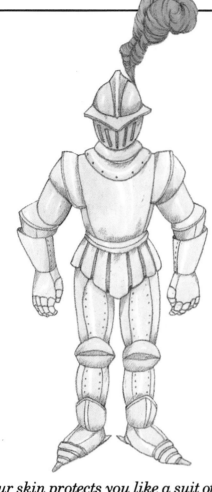

Your skin, the biggest part of you, stretches all over you like a tough but smooth suit of armor. It protects the body from dirt and germs, from the sun, and from temperatures that are too hot or too cold.

Skin is made up of two layers: the *epidermis* and the *dermis*. The epidermis is the thin top layer that you can see. That's the part that has the color or *pigment*. Your pigment determines the color of your skin. It also helps protect you from overexposure to the sun.

The outside layer of the epidermis is made up of old, dead skin. People lose dead skin bit by bit, in small flakes; snakes lose their skin all in one piece. Every time you dry yourself with a towel, you rub some skin off. Of course, new skin is growing underneath your old skin all the time, ready to take its place.

Your skin protects you like a suit of armor.

CROSS SECTION OF SKIN

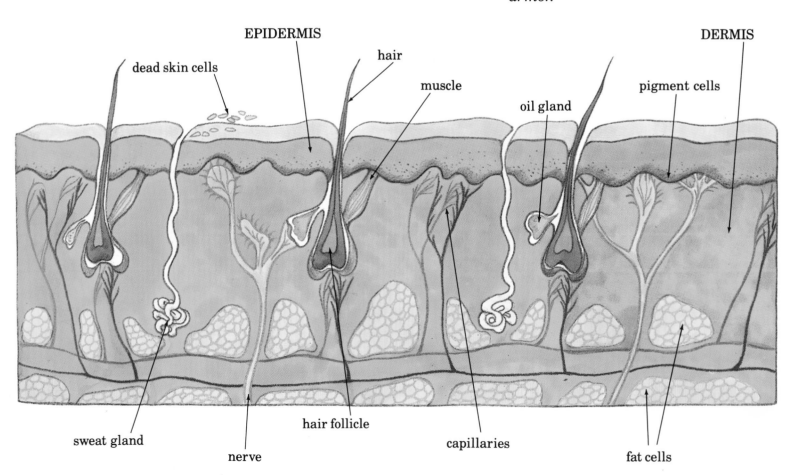

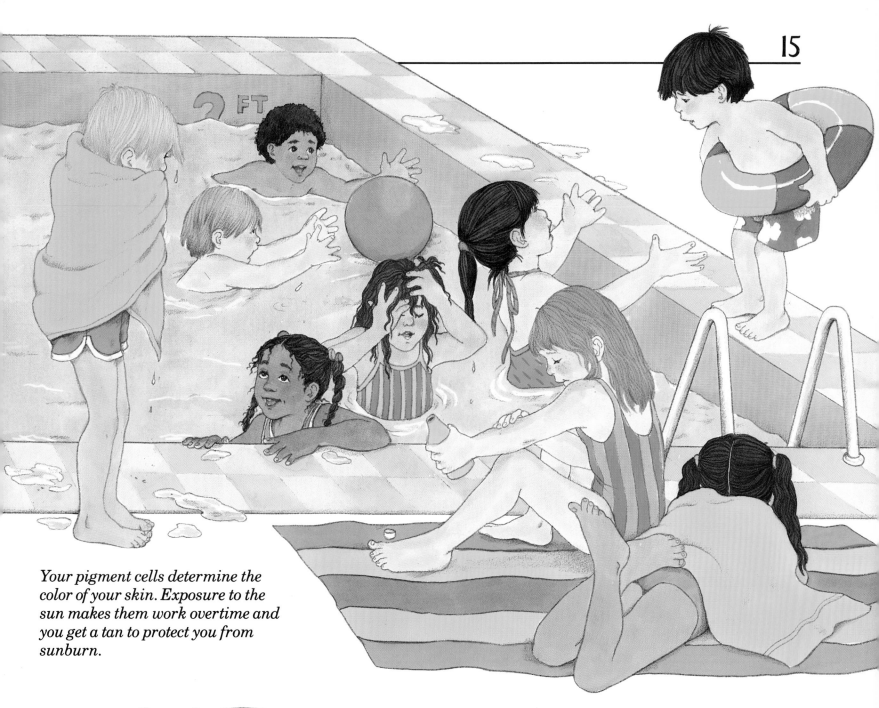

Your pigment cells determine the color of your skin. Exposure to the sun makes them work overtime and you get a tan to protect you from sunburn.

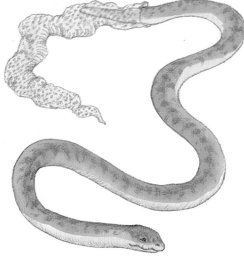

A snake sheds its dead skin cells all at once. Your dead skin cells rub off in little flakes.

Below the epidermis is the dermis, a thick layer of skin that is very much like a busy factory. It makes oil to keep your skin waterproof. Your skin also manufactures hair in tiny little pockets of skin called *follicles*. Attached to every follicle is a muscle. When you're cold, that muscle gets shorter and pulls on the hair to make it stand straight up. That's when your skin gets bumpy and people might say you have "goose bumps." Then you know it's time to get a sweater.

Fingernails and toenails, which are nothing more than a kind of hardened skin, are made deep within the dermis, too. There are no live nerves in your fingernails, toenails, or hair. That's why it doesn't hurt you when they are cut.

The Stomach, Intestines, and Digestion

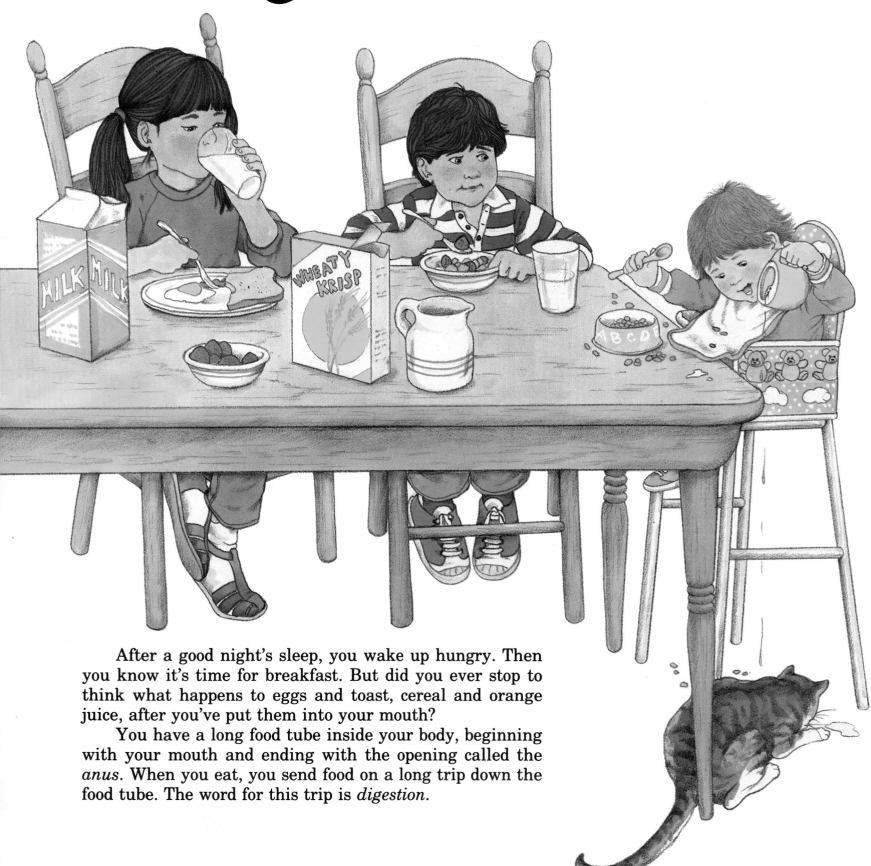

After a good night's sleep, you wake up hungry. Then you know it's time for breakfast. But did you ever stop to think what happens to eggs and toast, cereal and orange juice, after you've put them into your mouth?

You have a long food tube inside your body, beginning with your mouth and ending with the opening called the *anus*. When you eat, you send food on a long trip down the food tube. The word for this trip is *digestion*.

Before food can go anywhere, though, it must be broken up into small pieces. That's what your teeth are for. If food isn't chewed well enough, you could get a stomachache. The wet liquid in your mouth called spit or *saliva* helps get food ready for the trip down the food tube by making it smooth and soft. Saliva also helps change starches like bread into sugar needed by the body.

When you're all finished chewing, your tongue pushes the food to the back of your mouth. As you swallow, the muscles in your throat push the food again. Down it goes—through the part of your food tube called the *esophagus*.

As you chew, food is pushed by your tongue against the hard palate that forms the roof of your mouth. This process mixes the food with your saliva and starts your digestion working.

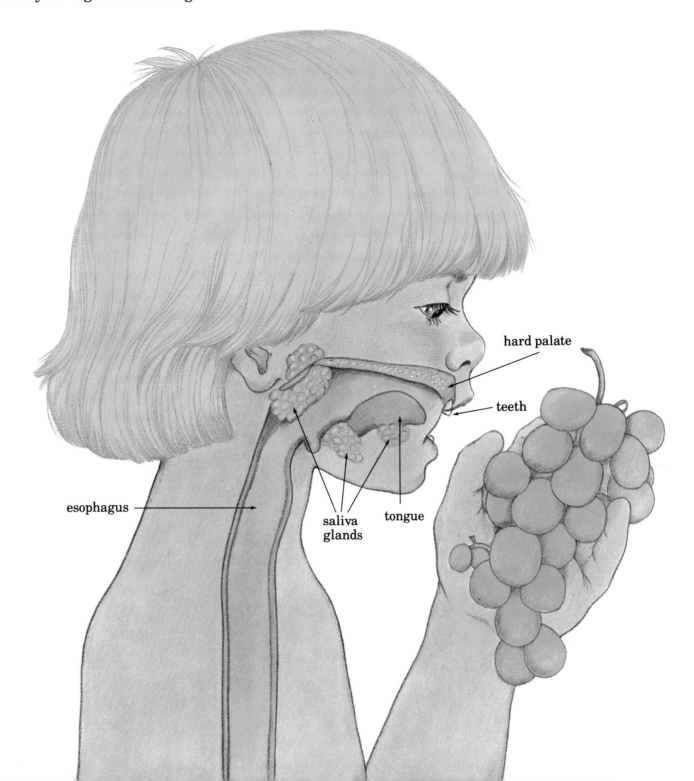

hard palate

teeth

esophagus

saliva glands

tongue

THE DIGESTIVE SYSTEM

Digestion starts in your mouth. From there the food travels down your esophagus to your stomach, where it is mashed up. As it passes through the small intestine, tiny villi gather up the nutrients your body needs. What the body does not need is pushed through the large intestine and out your anus as waste when you go to the bathroom.

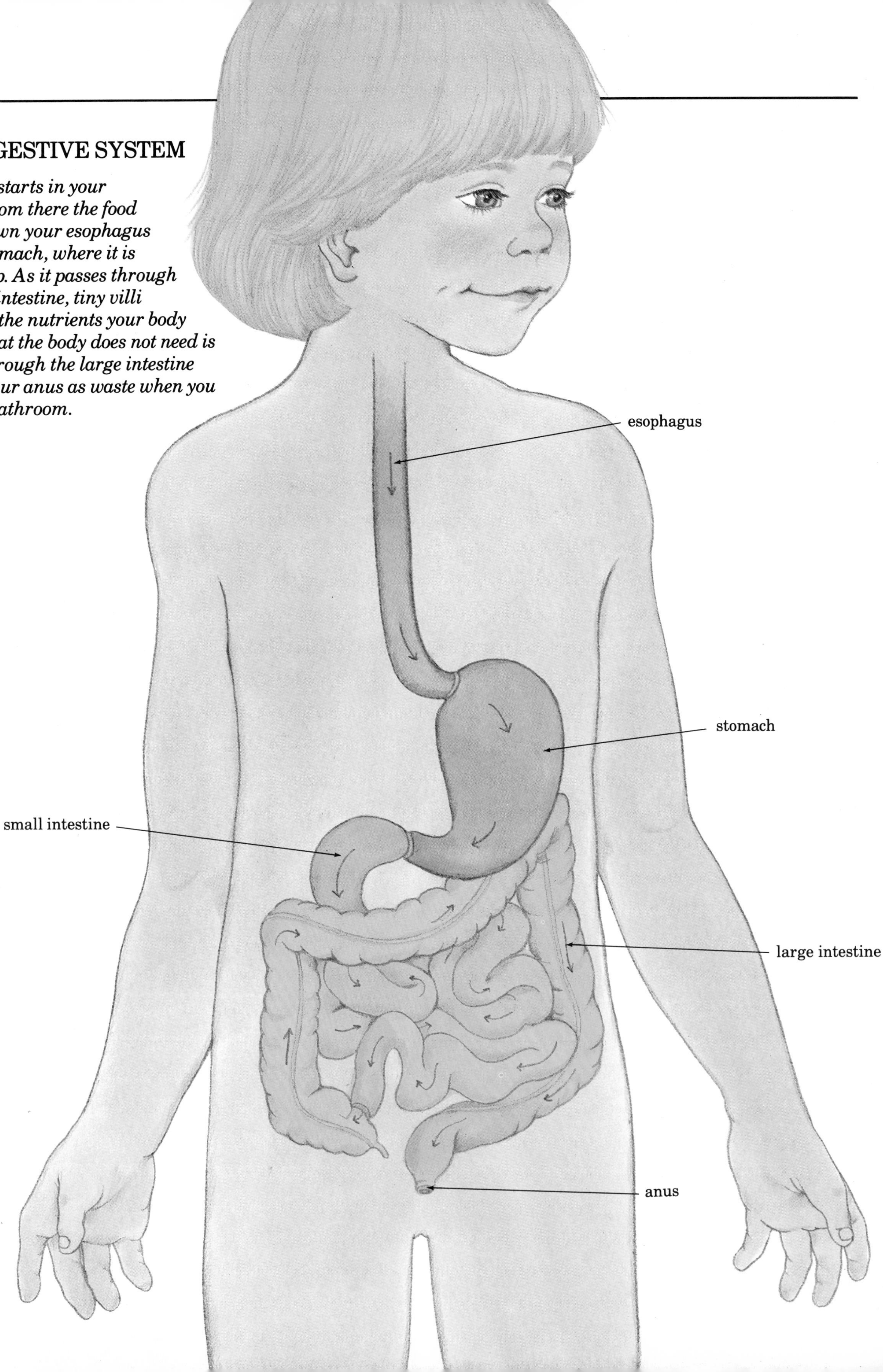

esophagus

stomach

small intestine

large intestine

anus

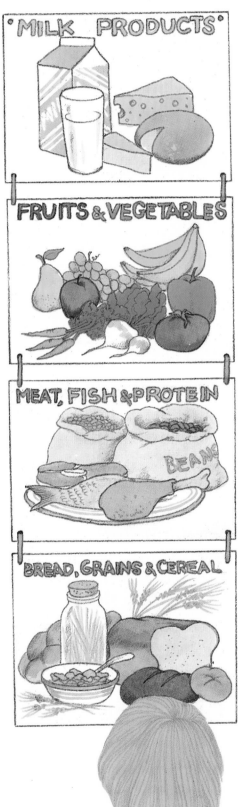

TODAY'S SPECIAL

MILK PRODUCTS

FRUITS & VEGETABLES

MEAT, FISH & PROTEIN

BREAD, GRAINS & CEREAL

Hairlike villi in your small intestine gather up the nutrients your body needs to keep working. The four groups of food that your body needs to remain healthy are shown to the left.

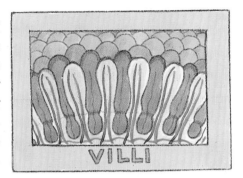

VILLI

The first stop is your stomach. Your stomach is a bag inside your body above your belly button or *navel*. When there's no food in it, your stomach is skinny like a balloon with no air in it. When it's full, it becomes fatter.

Your stomach works like a blender. It pushes bits of food around and around and around. It crushes and squeezes and mixes and mashes the food. Special stomach juices called *acids* help break down the food even more into a kind of soupy paste.

When your stomach has finished its part of the job of digesting food, your stomach muscles push the paste on to a new place called the *small intestine*. The small intestine is so long that it has to curl and twist like a snake in a basket just to fit inside of you. If you could somehow uncoil your small intestine to make it stand straight up, you'd have to be twenty feet tall to hold it all inside of you.

Your small intestine is filled with millions of tiny *villi*. Villi work like fingers to gather up all the parts of the food your body needs to keep on working. The rest is waste, the parts of food not needed by your body.

The muscles in the small intestine push the waste into a much thicker but shorter tube called the *large intestine*. It gets pushed farther and farther down to the end of the food tube until there is no place else for it to go. That's when you go to the bathroom and get rid of it all through the opening called your *anus*.

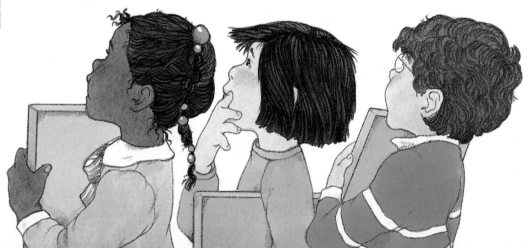

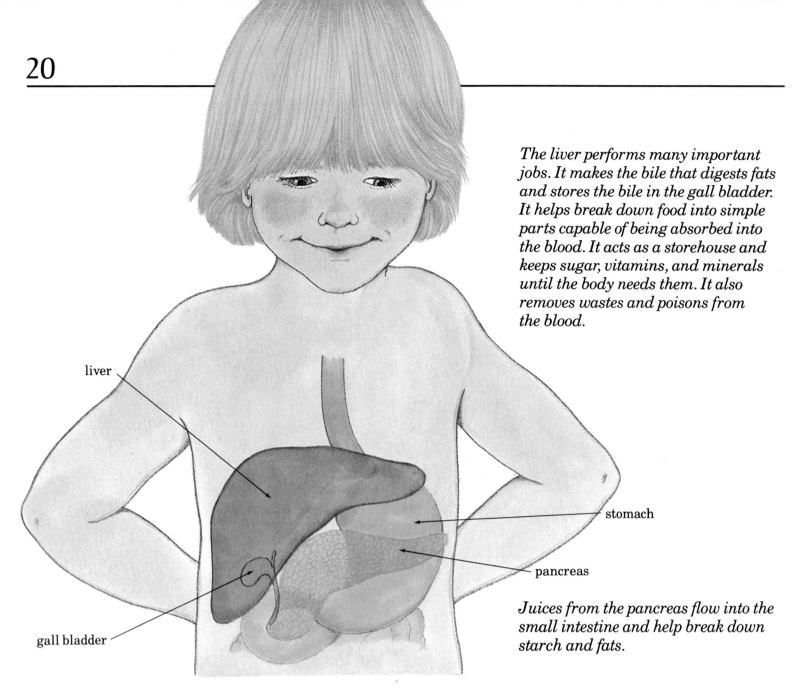

liver

gall bladder

stomach

pancreas

The liver performs many important jobs. It makes the bile that digests fats and stores the bile in the gall bladder. It helps break down food into simple parts capable of being absorbed into the blood. It acts as a storehouse and keeps sugar, vitamins, and minerals until the body needs them. It also removes wastes and poisons from the blood.

Juices from the pancreas flow into the small intestine and help break down starch and fats.

What happens to all the food that the villi in your small intestine have gathered up? These valuable bits of food pass into your capillaries. That is how the food that you ate gets into your blood. But before it can go to work for you, it has to go through an important cleaning and storing place called your *liver,* which is four times larger than your heart. The liver makes sure that your blood carries only the things that your body can use at that time. It takes out any extra vitamins and sugar you may have in your blood and stores them until you need them. Your liver also filters out harmful poisons from your blood.

Your blood is now ready to carry the digested food you need to every part of your body. Some of it will help you to move your arms, legs, fingers, and toes. Some will help you to grow new nails and hair; and some will help you to grow bigger and stronger.

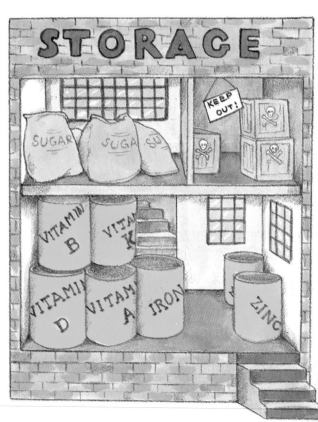

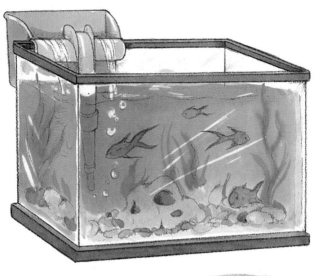

Once your blood has finished with this job, it carries the bits of used food and other wastes away. The blood carries these wastes to two special places called *kidneys*. Each kidney is five inches long and shaped something like a lima bean. Kidneys help get your blood ready for a new trip around your body. They work like the filter in a fish tank. The liquid that is cleaned out of your blood is called *urine*. Urine is stored in a balloonlike bag called the *bladder*. A tube leads from your bladder to the outside of your body. When your bladder is full, you feel uncomfortable. So off to the bathroom you go to get rid of all that yellow liquid that your body doesn't need.

THE URINARY SYSTEM

Like filters in fish tanks, the kidneys remove harmful wastes from the blood and send them down through tubes as urine to be stored in the bladder. When the bladder gets too full, you have to run off to the bathroom to get rid of all the urine.

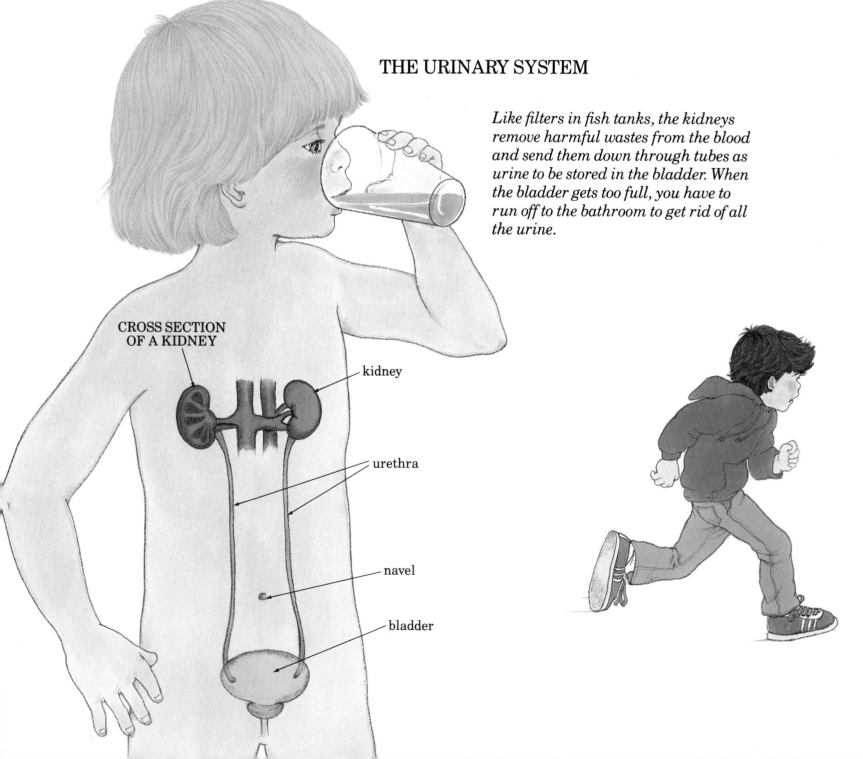

CROSS SECTION
OF A KIDNEY

kidney

urethra

navel

bladder

The Lungs and Breathing

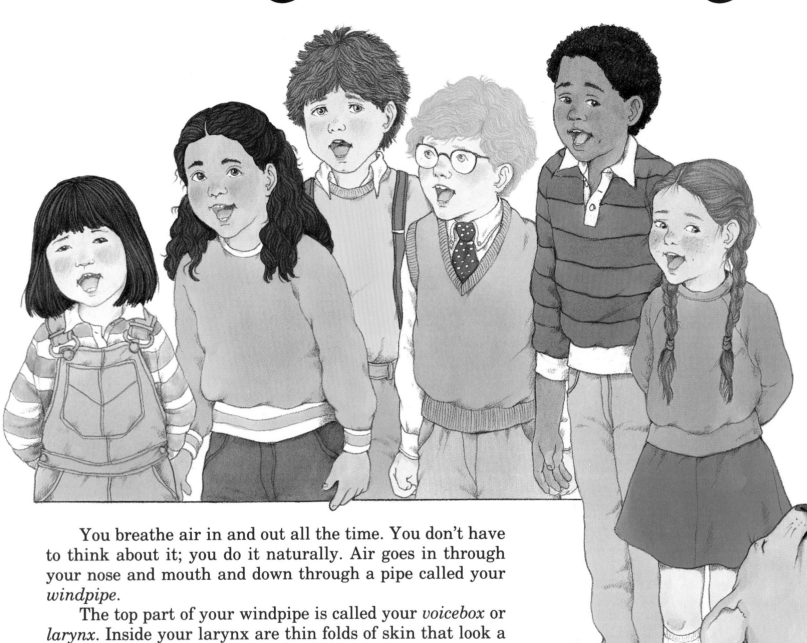

You breathe air in and out all the time. You don't have to think about it; you do it naturally. Air goes in through your nose and mouth and down through a pipe called your *windpipe*.

The top part of your windpipe is called your *voicebox* or *larynx*. Inside your larynx are thin folds of skin that look a bit like rubber bands. Those are your *vocal cords*. When you breathe out, you push air past them, causing them to flutter back and forth, or *vibrate*. The moving vocal cords create the sounds that are heard when you talk.

To make a sound, your vocal cords must first be stretched, just like rubber bands. If you pluck a rubber band, you get no sound at all. But if you stretch it beforehand, you may hear something. The muscles in your larynx do the same thing to your vocal cords. They can pull them tight to make your voice high and squeaky. They can pull them just a little to make your voice lower and smoother. Or they can completely relax. That's when your voice makes no sound at all.

THE RESPIRATORY SYSTEM

Air passes through your windpipe to your lungs. There tiny blood vessels gather up the oxygen in the air and your chest pushes out the used air to make room for a new lungful. The oxygen-bearing blood returns to the heart to begin its trip through your body. The heart then pushes old blood that has finished its trip into your lungs for a fresh supply of oxygen and the cycle begins again.

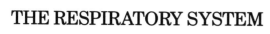

larynx

windpipe

lung

lung

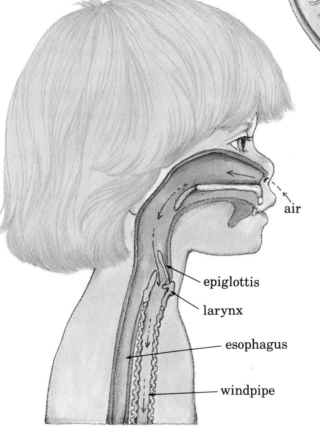

air

epiglottis

larynx

esophagus

windpipe

Your vocal cords are protected by your larynx. When you tighten your vocal cords, sound is produced by air passing across them on its way out of your lungs. When you swallow, the epiglottis shuts the opening to your windpipe, keeping food and liquid out of your lungs and allowing it to travel down your esophagus.

Your windpipe is like a hollow, upside-down tree trunk. It divides into two big branches, each of which ends up inside one of your *lungs.*

You have two lungs. When you are grown, each lung will be the size of a football. Lungs are inside your chest, one on each side of your heart.

Inside each of your lungs, the big branch of the windpipe divides into smaller and smaller branches; and each of these tiny branches ends in air sacs that work like balloons. When you breathe in, the branches carry air into the air sacs and fill up your lungs. Your chest gets bigger. While the sacs are filled with air, oxygen passes through them and into the tiny blood vessels nearby.

At the same time that your blood vessels are taking in new, clean air, used air passes from the blood vessels into the air sacs. So when you breathe out, you're getting rid of all that used-up air. Your chest gets smaller. Now it's time for a new breath. In, out, in, out—there's so much going on inside of you and you don't even have to think about it!

It's important to keep your air passageways clear. When you have a cold, a gluey liquid called *mucus* builds up inside your nose, throat, or air sacs. This makes it hard for you to breathe. Coughing is the way to get mucus out of your throat and lungs, and a sneeze is one of the best ways to clear it out of your nose.

The Brain and the Nervous System

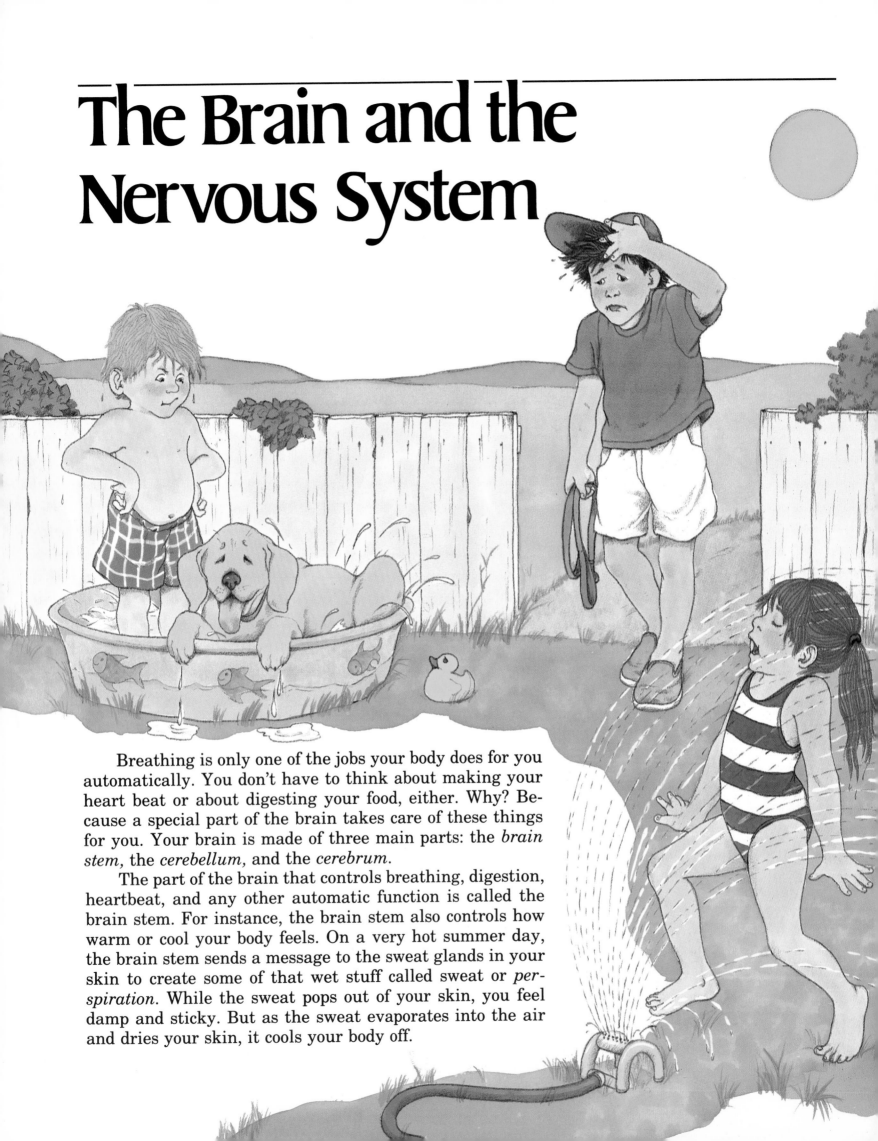

Breathing is only one of the jobs your body does for you automatically. You don't have to think about making your heart beat or about digesting your food, either. Why? Because a special part of the brain takes care of these things for you. Your brain is made of three main parts: the *brain stem,* the *cerebellum,* and the *cerebrum.*

The part of the brain that controls breathing, digestion, heartbeat, and any other automatic function is called the brain stem. For instance, the brain stem also controls how warm or cool your body feels. On a very hot summer day, the brain stem sends a message to the sweat glands in your skin to create some of that wet stuff called sweat or *perspiration.* While the sweat pops out of your skin, you feel damp and sticky. But as the sweat evaporates into the air and dries your skin, it cools your body off.

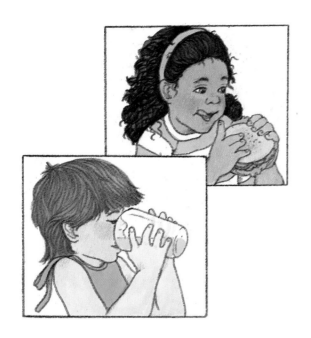

Sometimes the brain stem has to send a different kind of automatic message. When germs make you sick, the brain tells your sweat glands to stop working altogether. When that happens, you can't cool off, so your temperature goes up—you have a *fever*. A fever is a sign that your body is fighting to get rid of the germs that are making you sick. Since many germs can't live in hot places, a fever can help to kill them.

As the germs decrease, you start to get better. Since you don't need your fever anymore, your brain stem turns your sweat glands back on. You begin to perspire, and soon your temperature is back to normal again.

Your brain stem is responsible for all this and some other jobs, too. It makes you thirsty when your body needs water and hungry when your body needs food, and it makes you feel pain when you are injured.

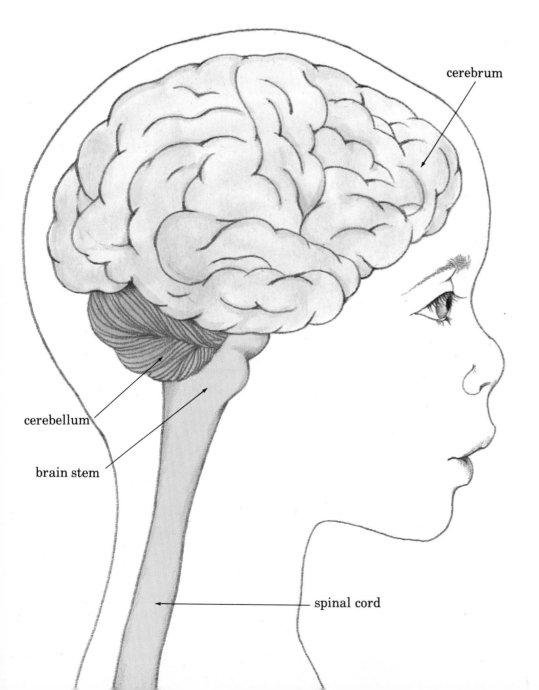

cerebrum

cerebellum

brain stem

spinal cord

Your brain consists of the brain stem, the cerebellum, and the cerebrum. The brain stem controls everything that happens automatically in your body. It makes your heart beat. It tells you when you are hungry or thirsty and when you feel pain. When you are sick, it causes a fever to help you fight germs.

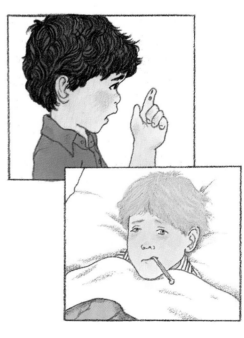

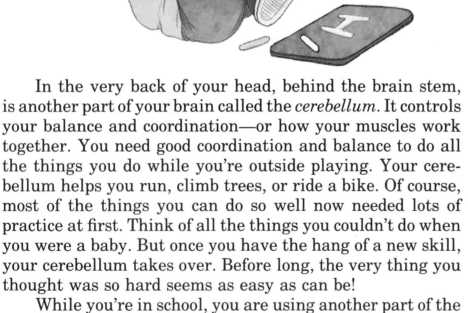

In the very back of your head, behind the brain stem, is another part of your brain called the *cerebellum*. It controls your balance and coordination—or how your muscles work together. You need good coordination and balance to do all the things you do while you're outside playing. Your cerebellum helps you run, climb trees, or ride a bike. Of course, most of the things you can do so well now needed lots of practice at first. Think of all the things you couldn't do when you were a baby. But once you have the hang of a new skill, your cerebellum takes over. Before long, the very thing you thought was so hard seems as easy as can be!

While you're in school, you are using another part of the brain called the *cerebrum*. As the biggest part of your brain, the cerebrum can store an amazing amount of information. It's where you do all your thinking, feeling, and remembering. Thinking can mean many things. Thinking is *learning* something new, such as how to write the letters of the alphabet. Thinking is *remembering* the letters so that you don't have to learn them again each time you want to use them. Thinking is *inventing*—putting the letters together in different ways to form words. Thinking is *choosing* to work with your letters instead of playing.

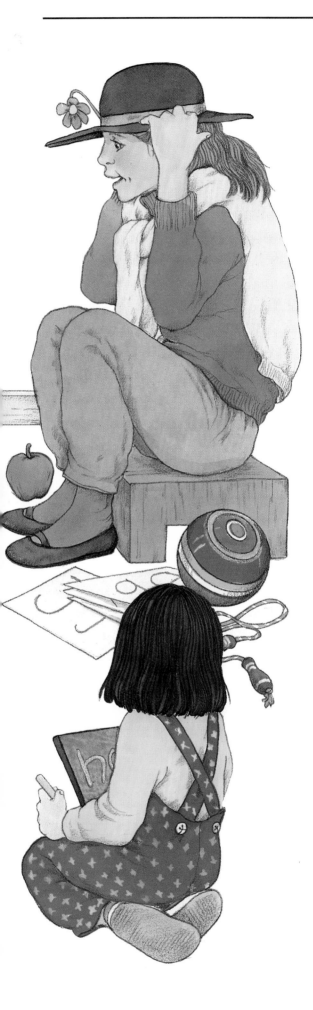

Nerve cells, or neurons, *receive information from your senses through feelers called* dendrites. *These sensations pass through the nucleus of the cell to pathways called* axons. *At the terminal of each axon the information is passed on to a new neuron until it reaches the brain and you hear, see, feel, taste, or smell.*

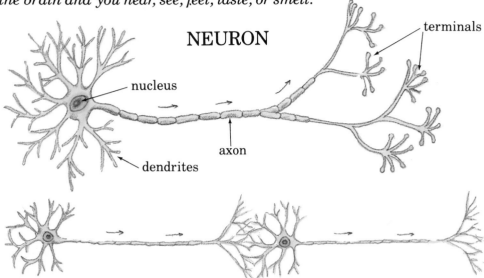

NEURON

terminals

nucleus

axon

dendrites

The cerebrum is also the feeling part of the brain. It controls two kinds of feelings: the *emotions* you feel on the inside, when you are happy, sad, angry, or scared; and the feelings that come to you from the outside through your senses, which are hearing, seeing, tasting, smelling, and touching.

The sense of *touch* comes to you through millions of tiny feelers that are right underneath your skin. They can tell you if the things you touch are hot or cold, hard or soft, sharp or smooth. All of these feelers are attached to long, thin message-carriers called *nerves*.

Nerves are made up of cells called *neurons*, connected to each other end to end, making pathways that lead to your brain. Some nerve pathways are short, like the ones that lead from your eye to your brain or from your ear to your brain. But you need a long pathway of nerves to get a message from your foot to your brain, since they are farther apart.

This long pathway of nerves is called the *spinal cord*. It is protected by a special part of your backbone called the *spinal column*. In fact, the spinal column protects most of the nerve pathways that run through your body. The spinal column is very much like a telephone cable with lots of wires running through it.

The nerves in your spinal cord are made of two kinds of fibers, or strands: those carrying messages to the brain and those carrying messages away from it. This message-carrying equipment—your brain and your spinal cord— make up what is known as your *central nervous system*.

THE NERVOUS SYSTEM

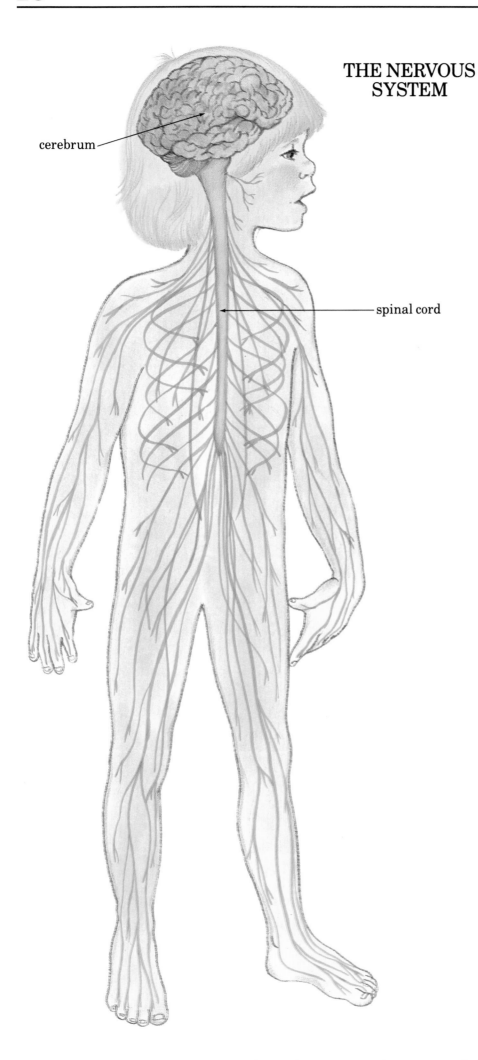

cerebrum

spinal cord

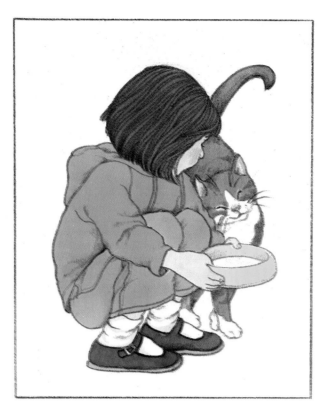

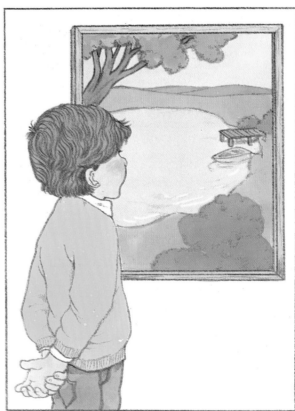

Your nervous system is like a giant computer, sending messages back and forth between your brain and the other parts of your body. The messages travel through your spinal cord to and from your cerebrum, which controls all the voluntary movements of your body and

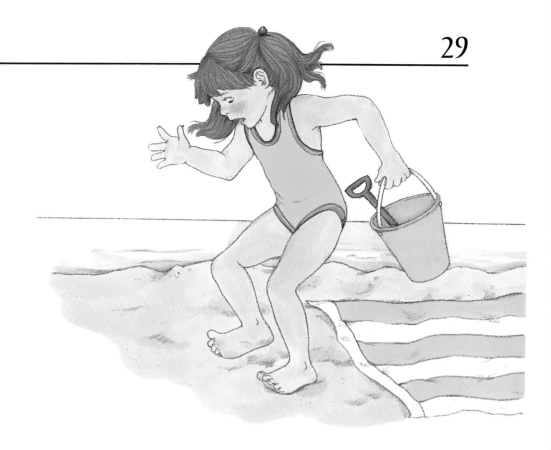

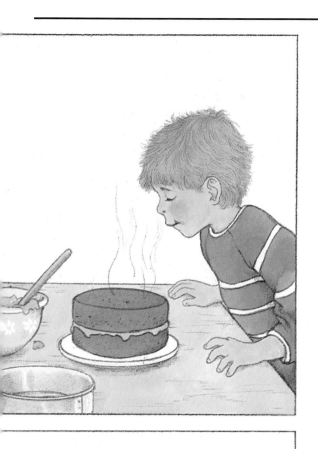

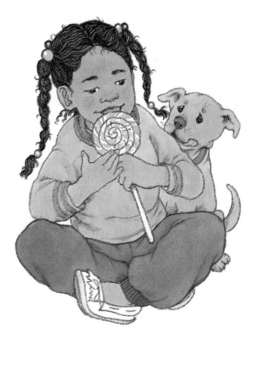

is responsible for thinking and learning. Messages from your sensory organs also travel through your spinal cord, and your cerebrum tells you what you are hearing, seeing, smelling, tasting, or feeling.

While the spinal cord carries messages back and forth from the brain to the lower part of the body, it also has another use. When you step barefoot on hot sand, your foot jerks back. This is called a *reflex action.* The pain message started in your toes, traveled through your legs, and caused a reflex action in your spinal cord, even before it reached the cerebrum. Your foot has jerked away even before your cerebrum lets you know what's wrong: the sand is too hot!

Now your brain (cerebrum) sends its own message down. Down, down, down it goes, through the spinal cord, until it reaches the muscles in your legs. What's the message? Stay on the beach blanket—and next time, better wear your sandals!

Your other senses help you gather information, too. Each one brings a message to your cerebrum from the world outside your body. Your memory helps you figure out what that message means. Memory is knowledge that has been tucked away for future use.

Your ears hear a meow. Your memory says "cat." Your eyes see a picture of water. Your memory says "lake." Your nose smells something good. Your memory says, "Could be cake!" Your tongue tastes something sweet. Your memory says "candy."

Your brain gets a message, figures it out, and tells your body what to do about it, all in the time it takes to blink an eye. It's the most wonderful computer ever built, and it fits right inside your head!

The Ear and the Eye

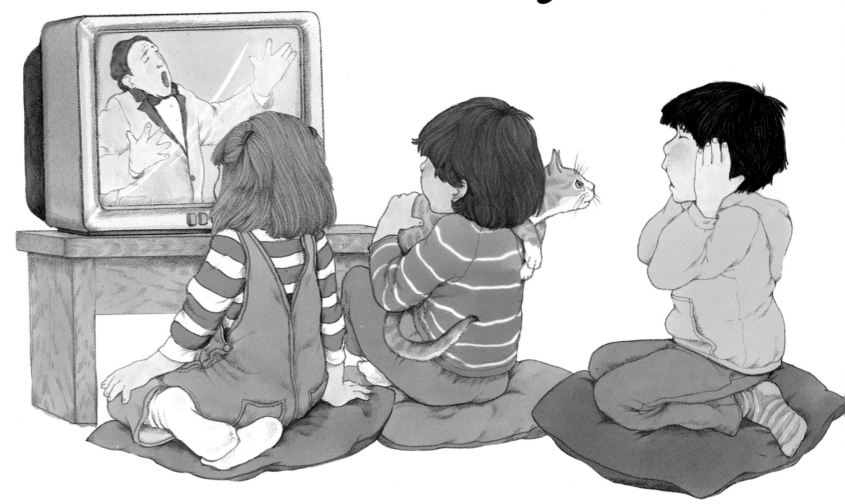

Ring . . . ring . . . ring . . . That could be the sound of a telephone—or a school bell. These are sounds that are heard as air moves back and forth, vibrating. The name for vibrating air is *sound waves.* Sound waves reach your outer ear (the part you can see) and then move on through a small tunnel called the *ear canal.*

Inside the ear canal is a thin sheet of skin called the *eardrum.* When sound waves reach it, your eardrum starts to vibrate, too.

There are three tiny little bones on the other side of your eardrum: the *hammer,* the *anvil,* and the *stirrup.* They pass sound waves along, one to the other, until they reach a larger, snail-shaped tube called the *cochlea.* The cochlea is lined with tiny, hairlike nerve endings and is filled with liquid. As soon as sound waves reach the cochlea, the liquid begins to shake, causing the nerve endings to vibrate. Vibrating nerve endings pass their message up a nerve pathway to the cerebrum. The cerebrum explains the sound to you, and you know just what it means.

HOW YOU HEAR

Sound waves pass into your ear through the ear canal and start your eardrum vibrating. Your tiny hammer, anvil, and stirrup bones pass the vibrations on to the cochlea and through it to your cerebrum.

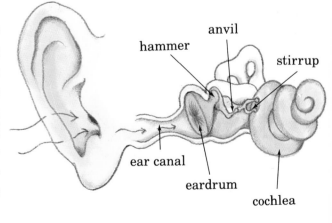

HOW YOU SEE

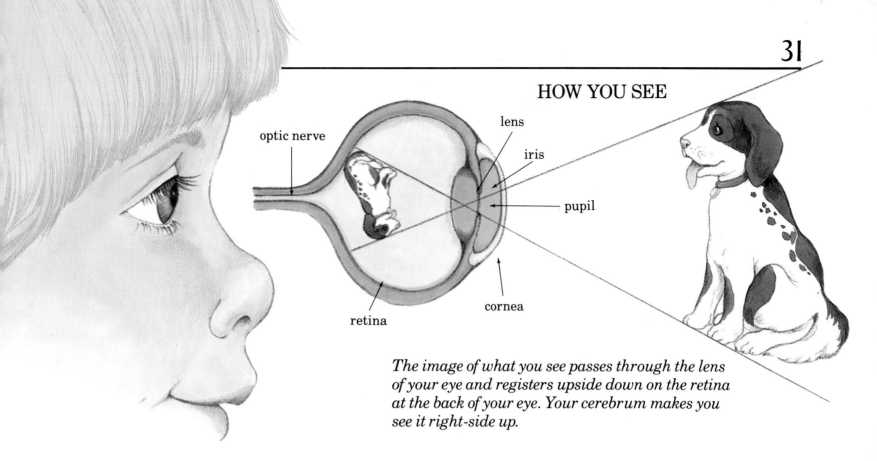

optic nerve

lens

iris

pupil

cornea

retina

The image of what you see passes through the lens of your eye and registers upside down on the retina at the back of your eye. Your cerebrum makes you see it right-side up.

Light passes through the pupil in the center of the iris. The less light there is, the wider the pupil opens.

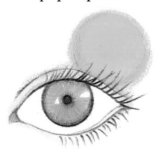

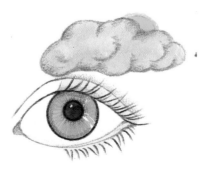

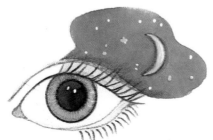

When you go outdoors on a bright, sunny day, it takes your eyes a while to adjust to all that sunlight. But light is what enters your eyes so that you can see. In the center of your eyeball is a little black circle called your *pupil*. The pupil is really a hole that lets the light in. Muscles in the *iris*, the colored part of your eye, make the pupil change its size depending on the lightness or darkness of where you are. When it's very dark, your pupil opens wider so that more light can come in. When it is very light, the pupil gets as small as a pencil point.

Your eye works like a camera. All of its parts—the lens, pupil, retina, and iris—work together to take pictures of things. The pictures are what you see.

The part of the eye called the *lens* is found right behind the pupil. It collects light rays and directs them to the back of your eye onto a kind of movie screen called the *retina*. The retina is covered with special nerve endings called *rods* and *cones*. When light shines on these nerve endings, they send a special message to the brain along a pathway called the *optic nerve*. In the cerebrum, this message is understood as a picture of what you are seeing.

The front part of your eyeball is a clear piece of skin that protects your eye like a windshield. It's called the *cornea*. To keep your eye clean and moist, you have a built-in watery fluid called tears. When you blink, your eyelid acts like a windshield wiper, washing all the dirt and germs out of your eyes. No movie camera ever invented, no matter how large, works quite as well as your own eyes.

Bones

Your bones form a framework on which your flesh hangs. The framework contains your vital organs, like the heart, lungs, and brain, and it protects them from harm.

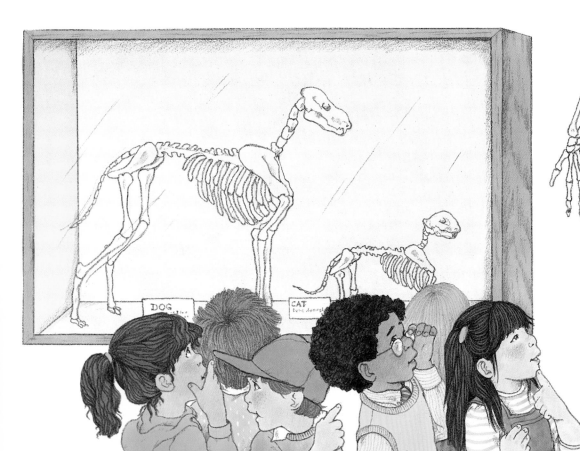

Bones are amazing, too. They give your body its shape. Without bones you might look something like a jellyfish! Since bones hold your whole body up, you would expect them to be pretty strong. They are. But the best part about bones is that, strong as they are, they don't weigh very much at all. That's why it's so easy for your muscles to move them around. Just think of all the things you can do with your body. If your bones were heavy, everything you did would be that much more difficult.

Your bones are alive. And like every other part of your body, they need food and oxygen to stay that way. If you are able to look at a bone closely, you will see that it is full of tiny holes. The holes are there so that blood vessels can bring food and oxygen into the bone where they're needed.

Your skeleton is made of different kinds of bones—long bones, short bones, and flat bones.

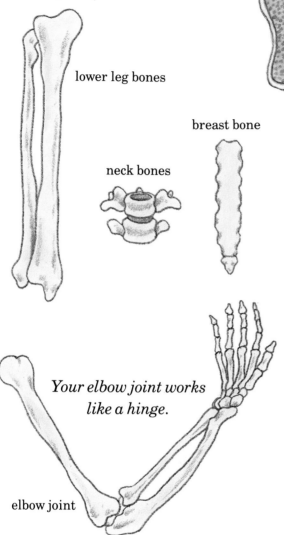

lower leg bones

breast bone

neck bones

Your elbow joint works like a hinge.

elbow joint

When you break a bone, the doctor keeps it in place with a cast until the bone grows together and is mended.

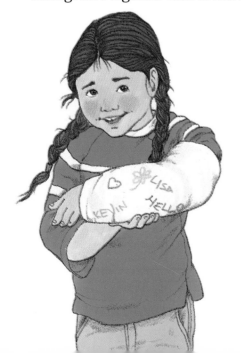

The part of a bone that is not hollow contains living bone cells.

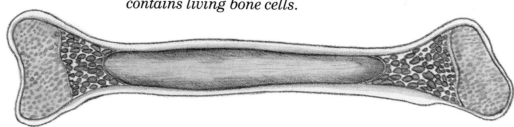

The insides of your bones are hollow. That's what makes them so light. Some of the spaces inside your bones are taken up by a material called *marrow*. The marrow parts of certain bones work day and night to make red blood cells and some white cells—something your blood always needs in fresh supply. The brand-new blood cells find their way into the blood through tiny capillaries that are woven through the bone.

You have lots of bones—about 206 of them—and there are different types of bones for different movements. Some movements, such as walking and throwing, need *long bones,* like the ones within your arms and legs. The biggest bone you have is the *femur,* better known as your thighbone.

Other movements, such as writing or tapping your foot, need only *short bones,* like the ones within your wrists and ankles. The smallest bone in your body is that tiny little bone in your ear called the stirrup. Isn't it remarkable that a bone so small can help you hear a sound as big as thunder?

Your breastbone, skull, and ribs are your *flat bones.* They protect all those very important soft parts of you, like your heart, lungs, and brain.

The place where one bone connects with another bone is called a *joint.* There are joints between the bones in your back. That's why you can bend in many directions. Your knees and elbows are joints, too. Can you think of any other places that you have joints? Think of all the joints you need for special movements, such as twisting, turning, and bending.

You have to fall quite hard to break a bone, so most of us never find out what it's like to break an arm or a leg. But suppose you do break an arm? A doctor will carefully fit the pieces back together, then put a plaster cast around your arm to make sure that the pieces don't move out of place. While your arm is in the cast, the living parts of the bone will form immature bone cells called *callus.* Callus fills in the spaces between the broken ends like a glue so that they'll stick together. By the time the doctor is ready to take the cast off, your broken bone will have mended, and there is brand-new, strong bone where the callus used to be!

Muscles

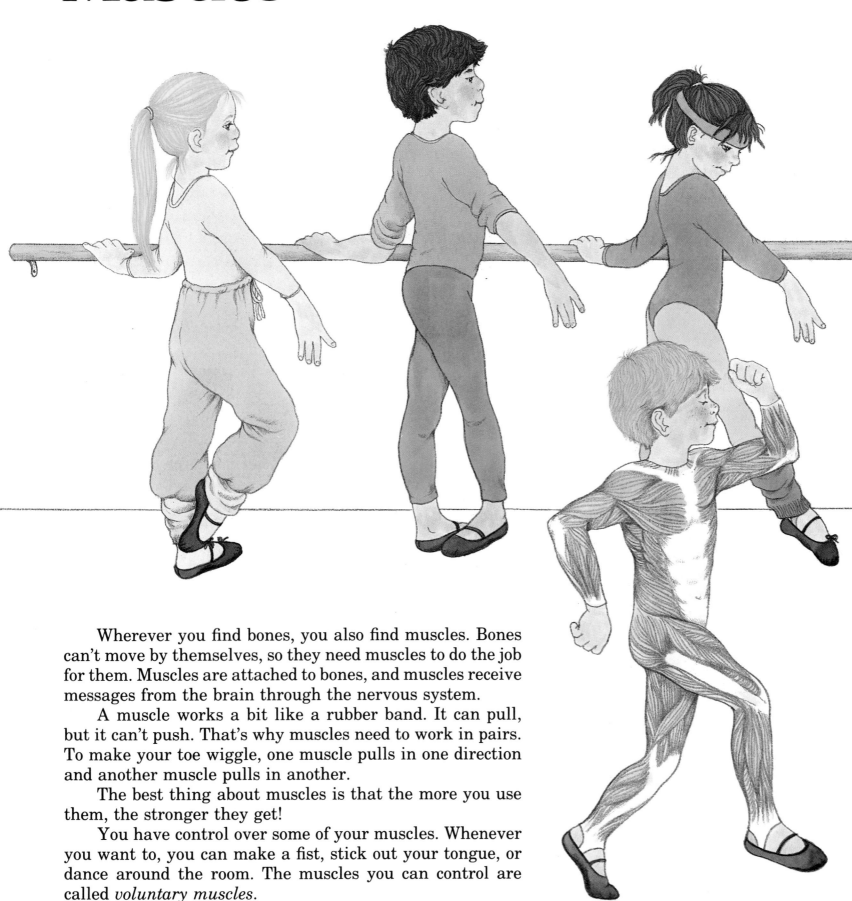

Wherever you find bones, you also find muscles. Bones can't move by themselves, so they need muscles to do the job for them. Muscles are attached to bones, and muscles receive messages from the brain through the nervous system.

A muscle works a bit like a rubber band. It can pull, but it can't push. That's why muscles need to work in pairs. To make your toe wiggle, one muscle pulls in one direction and another muscle pulls in another.

The best thing about muscles is that the more you use them, the stronger they get!

You have control over some of your muscles. Whenever you want to, you can make a fist, stick out your tongue, or dance around the room. The muscles you can control are called *voluntary muscles*.

INVOLUNTARY MUSCLES

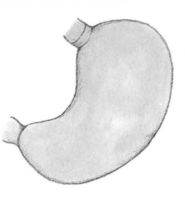

heart   stomach

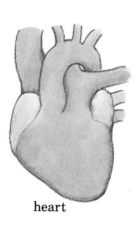

The iris in your eye automatically gets smaller to keep out bright light.

Muscles attached to hair follicles in the skin automatically cause goose bumps when you are cold.

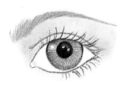

But some muscles work on their own. Your heart is a good example. It keeps beating even when you're sleeping. Its muscles are called *involuntary*. Other involuntary muscles include those in the iris that react to light quickly, and those attached to hair follicles that cause you to get goose bumps.

Did you know that you have sixteen muscles in your face just to show people how you feel? When you're happy, your brain sends a message to one set of muscles to lift up the corners of your mouth. Then, when you are finished smiling, your brain tells another set of muscles to pull them back down again to their normal place. The next time you look in the mirror, see how many "faces" your muscles can help you make.

Voluntary muscles are those muscles over which you have control. You use them to make faces, walk, run, and dance. Involuntary muscles keep working automatically whether you tell them to or not. There is no way you can tell your heart to stop beating.

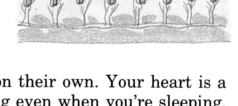

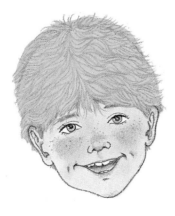

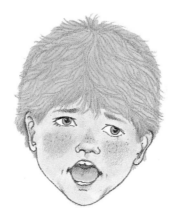

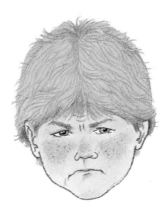

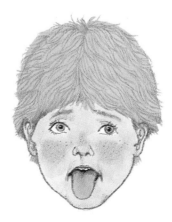

Heredity

While you're looking in the mirror, take an extra minute or two to admire yourself. Is your hair curly or straight? Do you have dimples or freckles? What color are your eyes? Do you ever wonder why you look the way you do?

You look the way you do because of *genes*. Genes are like the ingredients in a recipe. Put them all together in the right order and in the right amount and you get the recipe for you.

Every part of you is made up of tiny living things called *cells*. They're so tiny that you need a microscope to see them. And tucked away in the center of every cell in your body are tiny threads called *chromosomes* that carry even tinier things called *genes*. The cells that make up your bones look different from the cells that make up your skin, because your genes tell your cells exactly how to grow. They say, "Bones, be hard. Skin, be soft. Eyes, be blue," or "green," or "brown," or "black." There are genes for almost everything about you. You have special genes for your voice, for your height, for the shape of your ears, nose, and mouth, and even for your fingernails.

Your body is made of millions and millions and millions of cells. In the center of each are chromosomes carrying tiny genes. The genes tell each cell just how to grow to be a nerve cell, a muscle cell, or whatever kind of cell it is going to be.

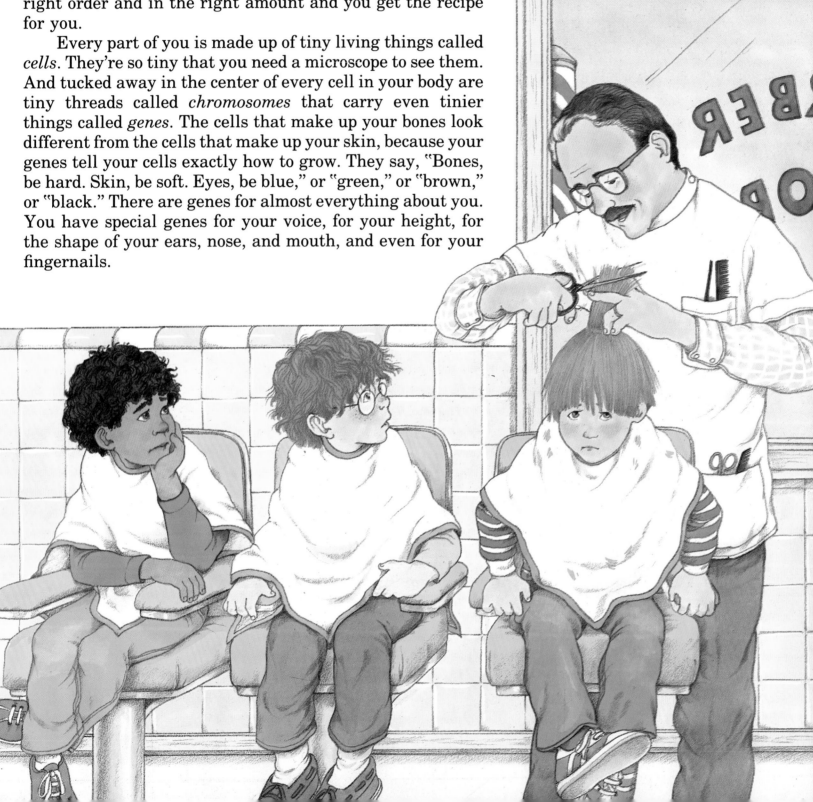

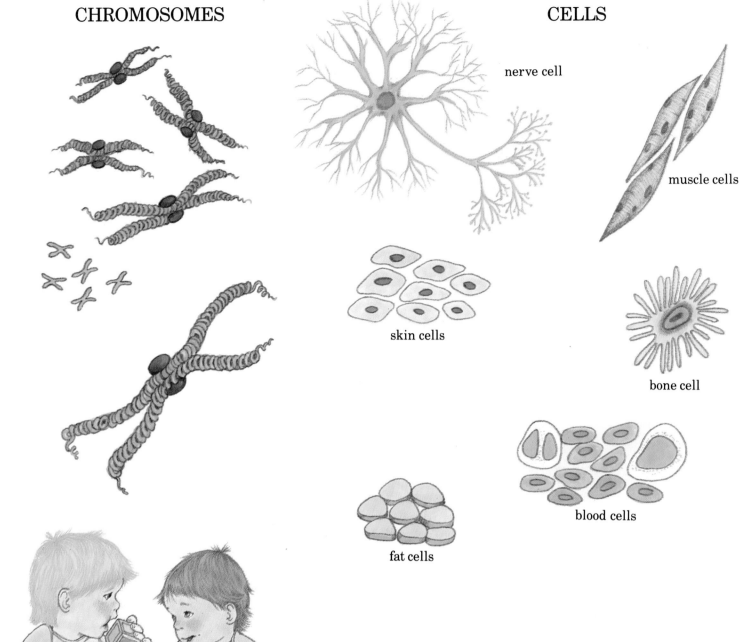

CHROMOSOMES

CELLS

nerve cell

muscle cells

skin cells

bone cell

blood cells

fat cells

If the father's baby-making cell contains an x-chromosome, the baby will be a girl. If it contains a y-chromosome, it will be a boy.

Each of us starts out when a special baby-making cell from a father joins a special baby-making cell from a mother. The father's cell has half of all the genes needed to make a new person and the mother's cell has the other half. These genes are found on the chromosomes at the center of the baby-making cells. There are 23 chromosomes from Mom and 23 chromosomes from Dad, all paired up.

One pair of these chromosomes makes the baby a girl or boy. The baby-making cell of the mother has what's called an *x-chromosome,* but the baby-making cell of the father may have an x-chromosome or something called a *y-chromosome.* The father's cell is the one that is able to make the baby a boy or a girl. If that cell turns out to have an x-chromosome, the baby will be a girl; if it has a y-chromosome, the baby will be a boy.

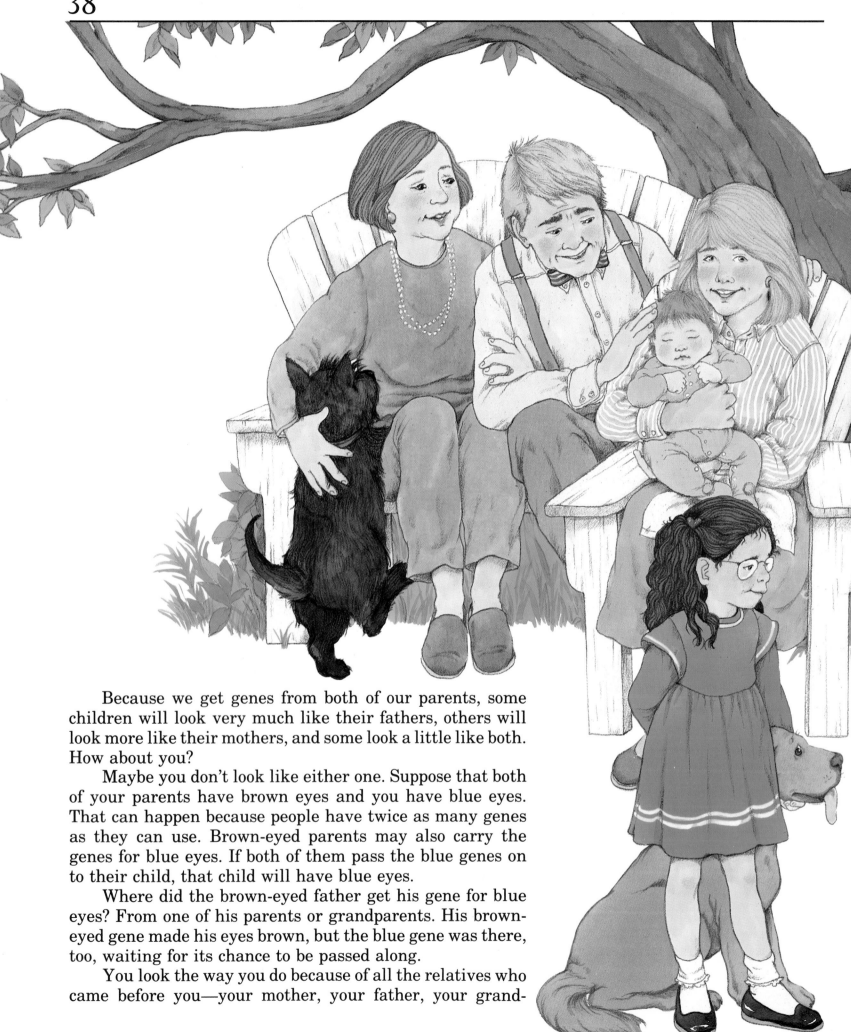

Because we get genes from both of our parents, some children will look very much like their fathers, others will look more like their mothers, and some look a little like both. How about you?

Maybe you don't look like either one. Suppose that both of your parents have brown eyes and you have blue eyes. That can happen because people have twice as many genes as they can use. Brown-eyed parents may also carry the genes for blue eyes. If both of them pass the blue genes on to their child, that child will have blue eyes.

Where did the brown-eyed father get his gene for blue eyes? From one of his parents or grandparents. His brown-eyed gene made his eyes brown, but the blue gene was there, too, waiting for its chance to be passed along.

You look the way you do because of all the relatives who came before you—your mother, your father, your grand-

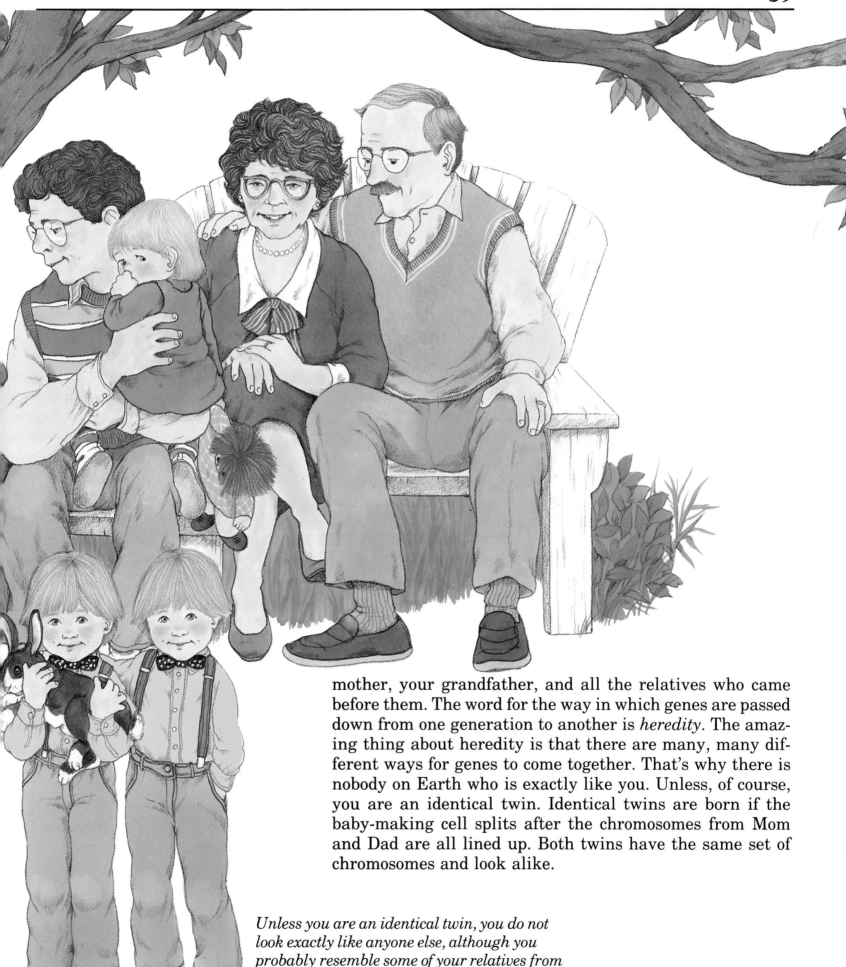

mother, your grandfather, and all the relatives who came before them. The word for the way in which genes are passed down from one generation to another is *heredity*. The amazing thing about heredity is that there are many, many different ways for genes to come together. That's why there is nobody on Earth who is exactly like you. Unless, of course, you are an identical twin. Identical twins are born if the baby-making cell splits after the chromosomes from Mom and Dad are all lined up. Both twins have the same set of chromosomes and look alike.

Unless you are an identical twin, you do not look exactly like anyone else, although you probably resemble some of your relatives from whom you inherited your genes.

The Reproductive System

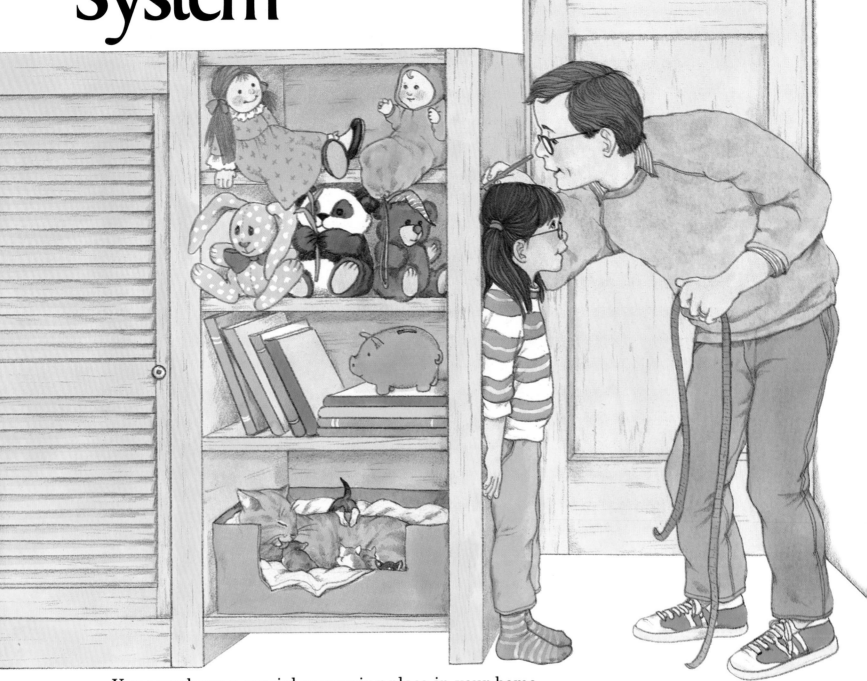

You may have a special measuring place in your home to keep a record of how tall you are. It's fun to see, by comparing the marks or notches on a wall, how many inches you have grown from year to year.

You probably already know that you are growing all of the time. You can tell when all of a sudden the sleeves of your favorite outfit seem a little too short, or when a toe starts to poke out through your sneaker. But did you know that you were growing even before you were born?

Your father's sperm cell united with your mother's egg cell to form the new cell that was to become you. That cell kept dividing until at last you were you.

FATHER'S BABY-MAKING CELL

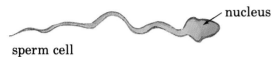

sperm cell   nucleus

MOTHER'S BABY-MAKING CELL

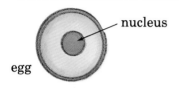

nucleus

egg

CELL DIVISION

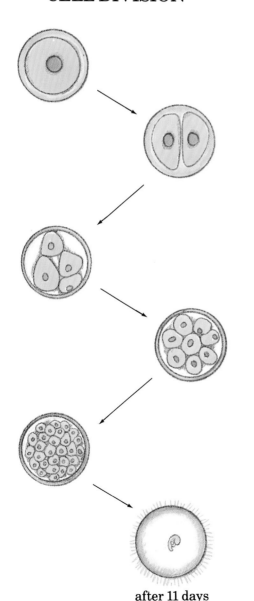

after 11 days

You started out as a tiny speck inside your mother. This speck was the egg that was half the recipe for you, and it was there inside of your mother when your mother was born. If you are a girl, you already have all of the eggs you'll ever need to make babies of your own someday. They're stored deep inside of you in two round little pouches called *ovaries*.

But that egg that made you had only half of what was needed to make a baby, so it stayed inside your mother's ovary with many other eggs. The eggs waited and waited for a chance to take a trip down one of two special passageways called *fallopian tubes*.

Finally it was time for your egg to make its trip. As it moved down the tube, it met another tiny speck called a *sperm*. The sperm came from your father and it had within it the recipe for the other half of you. The sperm joined the egg and something truly wonderful happened! Together the sperm and the egg became a single cell—the brand-new life that was you!

This single cell had the mysterious power to make more cells. The new cell divided into two; then these two divided to make four. They continued dividing until there were many cells that all clung together like soapsuds in a bubble.

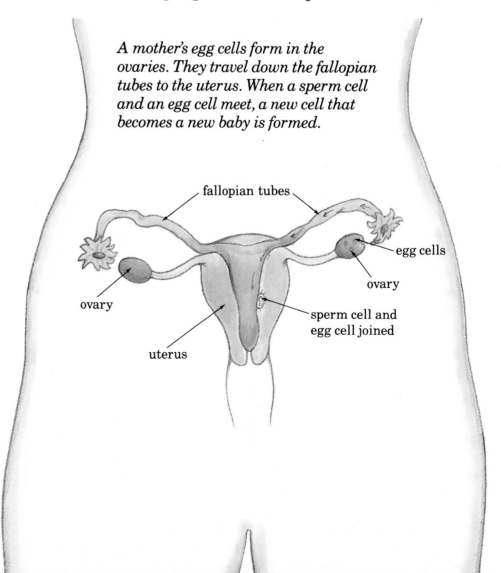

A mother's egg cells form in the ovaries. They travel down the fallopian tubes to the uterus. When a sperm cell and an egg cell meet, a new cell that becomes a new baby is formed.

fallopian tubes

egg cells

ovary

ovary

sperm cell and egg cell joined

uterus

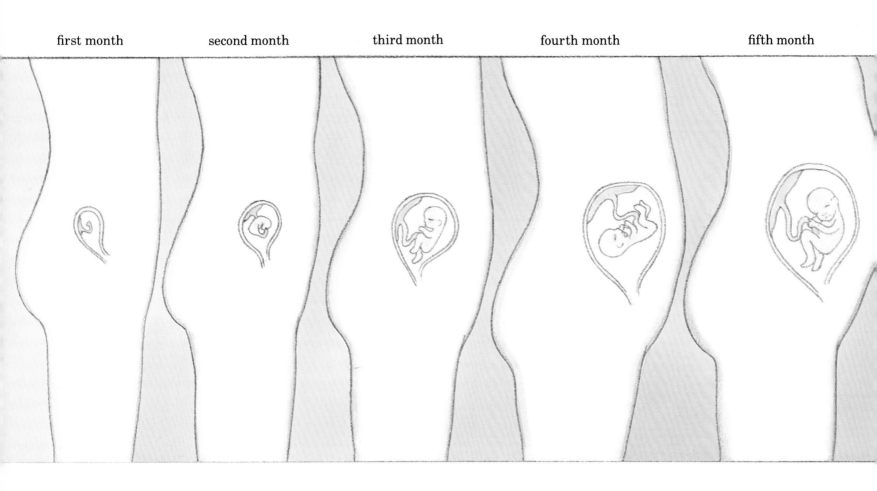

You grew bigger every month you spent in your mother's body as an embryo. You were only as big as the eraser on a pencil by the end of the first month. By the ninth month you were a full-grown baby.

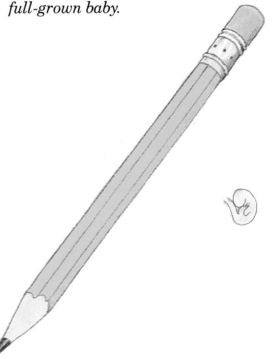

The whole time that they were dividing, the cells kept on moving down the fallopian tube tunnel until they reached the special baby-growing place called the *uterus*. When they got to the uterus, they attached themselves to one of its walls and continued to grow. Soon a protective sac, called the *placenta,* grew around the cells like a balloon, which soon filled with a warm liquid to make a safe, watery cocoon for the cells to grow in. Scientists call these growing cells an *embryo.*

The embryo stayed there and continued to grow for the nine months it takes to make a baby. The food your mother ate fed you, too, while you were an embryo. It flowed from her to you through a tube that was connected to your middle. This tube is called the *umbilical cord.*

By the end of the first month of life, you were just about the size of the eraser on the end of a pencil. Little by little you grew. Soon the doctor could hear your heartbeat when he placed the stethoscope on your mother's tummy. The bud-like nubs on either side of your body began to unfold into

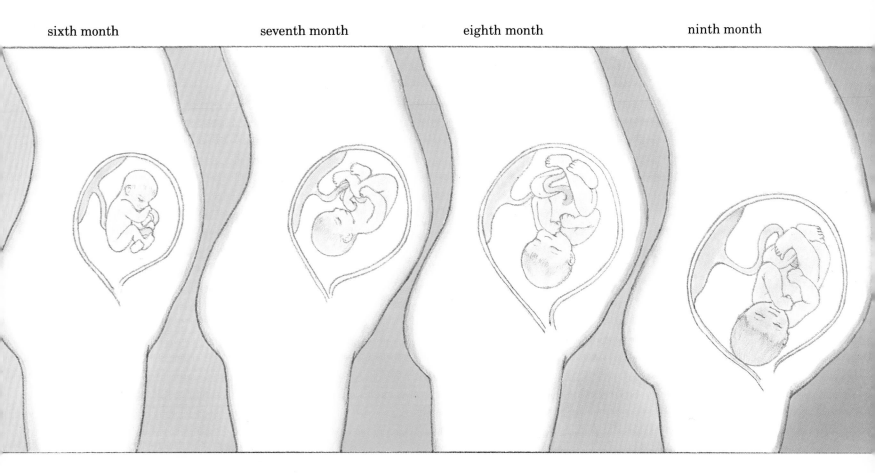

sixth month   seventh month   eighth month   ninth month

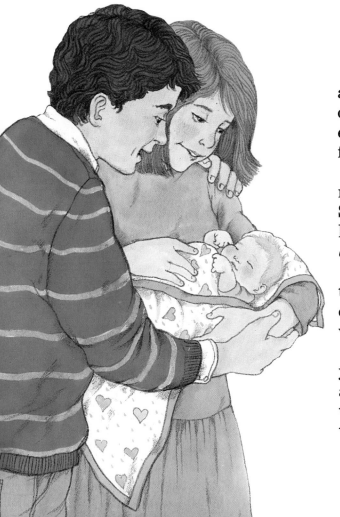

arms. The stubs at the end of your body took on the shape of legs, and by the fourth month of your life, you started to exercise them by giving little kicks that your mother could feel.

Your mother's uterus expanded as you grew until the ninth month, when there was no more room for it to grow. So the walls of the uterus began to squeeze and squeeze. At last they pushed you through the tunnel that is called the *birth canal,* and out you came into the world!

The doctor then cut the umbilical cord that joined you to your mother and kept you nourished while you lived inside of her. The part that was left eventually healed, and that is where your belly button is today.

When your parents brought you home from the hospital, you slept most of the time. But you've grown a lot since then and now you don't need to sleep nearly so much. It's a good thing, too, because there are so many other more interesting things to do in a day.

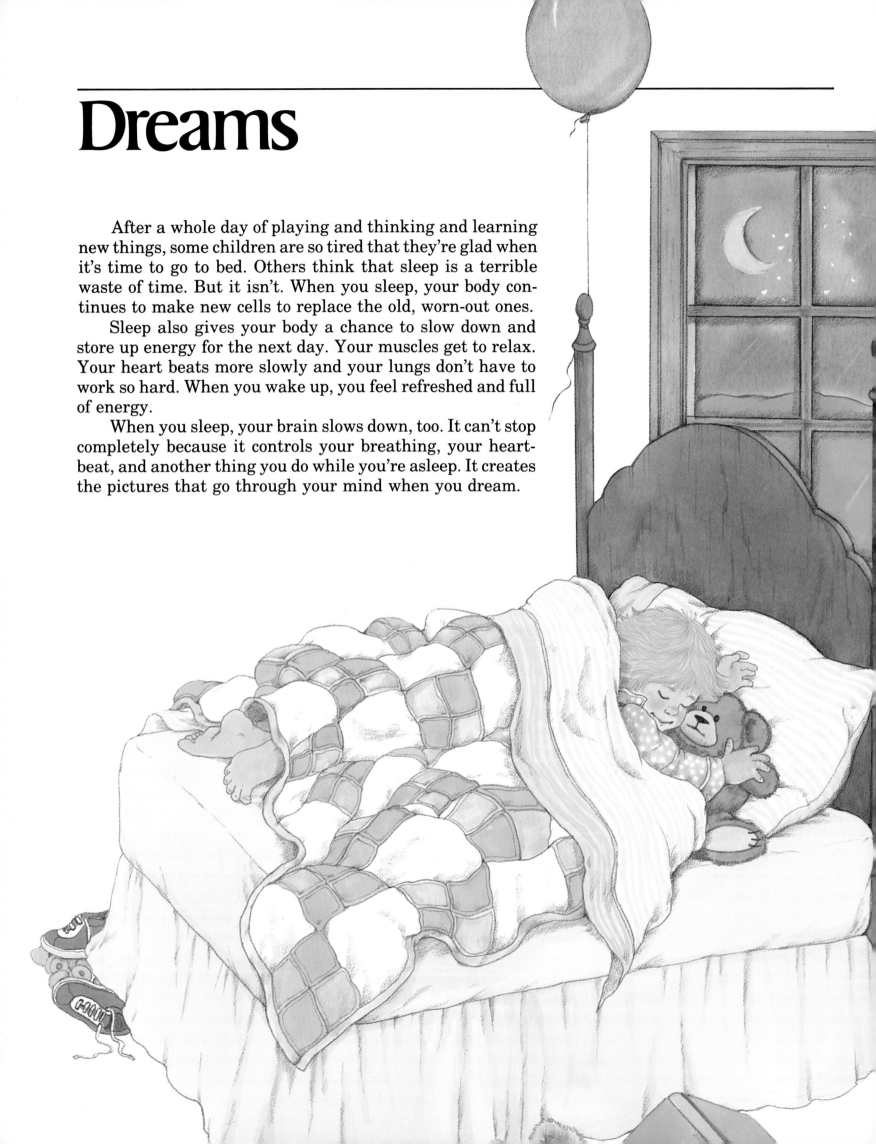

Dreams

After a whole day of playing and thinking and learning new things, some children are so tired that they're glad when it's time to go to bed. Others think that sleep is a terrible waste of time. But it isn't. When you sleep, your body continues to make new cells to replace the old, worn-out ones.

Sleep also gives your body a chance to slow down and store up energy for the next day. Your muscles get to relax. Your heart beats more slowly and your lungs don't have to work so hard. When you wake up, you feel refreshed and full of energy.

When you sleep, your brain slows down, too. It can't stop completely because it controls your breathing, your heartbeat, and another thing you do while you're asleep. It creates the pictures that go through your mind when you dream.

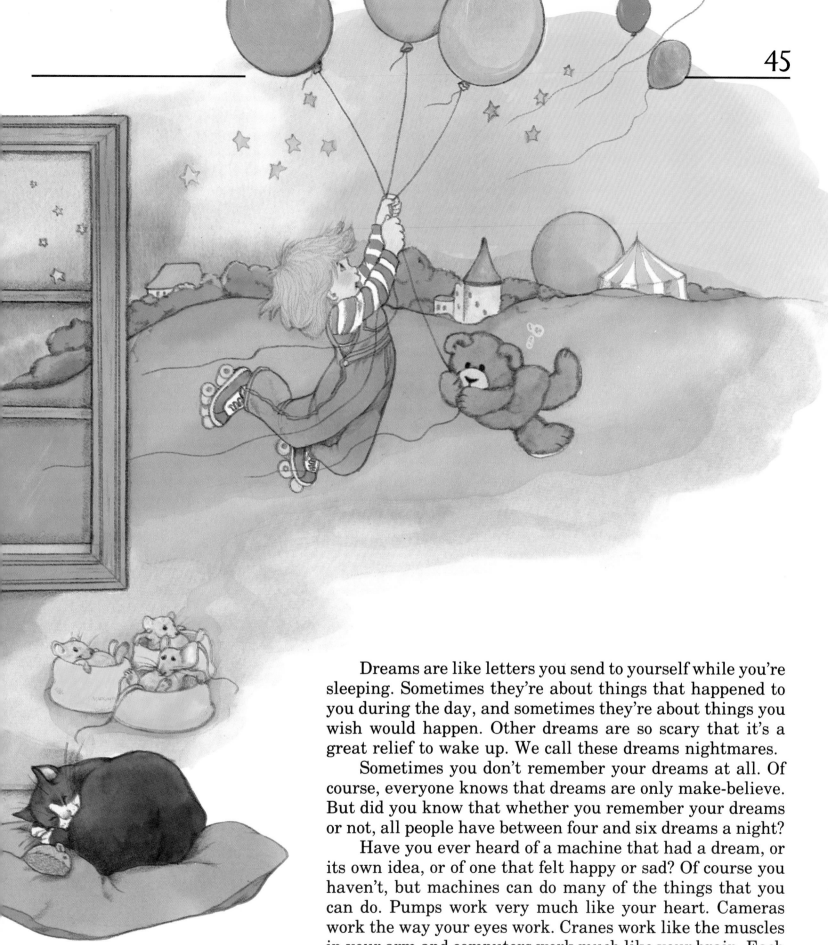

Your brain works even while you are sleeping. It sends messages to you in the form of dreams.

Dreams are like letters you send to yourself while you're sleeping. Sometimes they're about things that happened to you during the day, and sometimes they're about things you wish would happen. Other dreams are so scary that it's a great relief to wake up. We call these dreams nightmares.

Sometimes you don't remember your dreams at all. Of course, everyone knows that dreams are only make-believe. But did you know that whether you remember your dreams or not, all people have between four and six dreams a night?

Have you ever heard of a machine that had a dream, or its own idea, or of one that felt happy or sad? Of course you haven't, but machines can do many of the things that you can do. Pumps work very much like your heart. Cameras work the way your eyes work. Cranes work like the muscles in your arm and computers work much like your brain. Each is quite good at doing the *one* thing it was made to do. But your body can do all of these things and more. Now that you know so much about the way your insides work, don't you agree that you are pretty special?

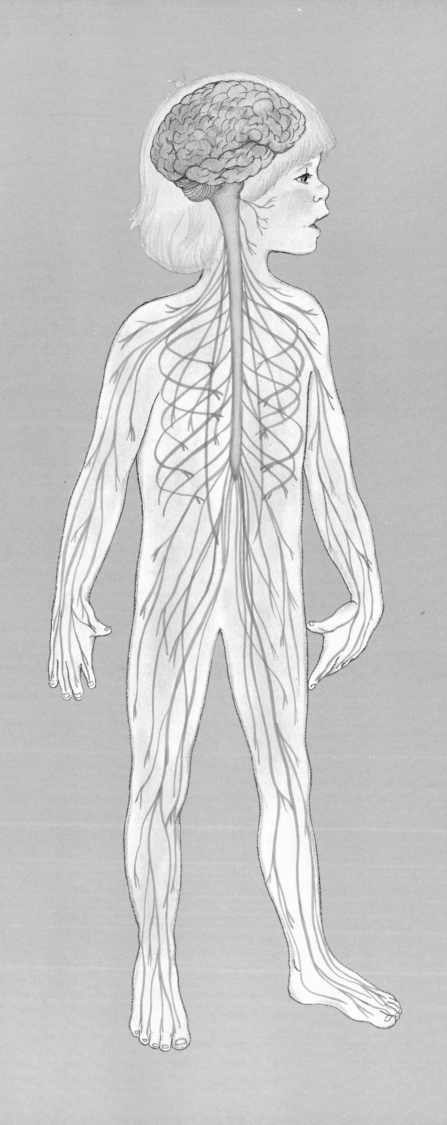